FIVE-MINUTE

BEAUTIFUL

NAILS

FIVE-MINUTE

BEAUTIFUL

NAILS

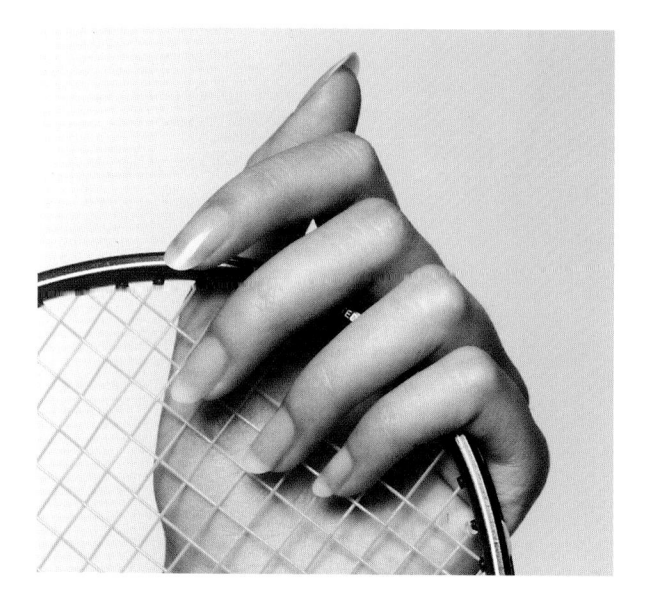

TANYA BODEN

TIGER BOOKS INTERNATIONAL
LONDON

Conceived and produced by Breslich & Foss Ltd., London

Photography by Nigel Bradley
Illustrations by Marilyn Leader
Text written in collaboration with Laura Wilson
Designed by Clare Finlaison
Original design by Lisa Tai

This edition published in 1997 by
Tiger Books International PLC, Twickenham

ISBN 1-85501-896-9

Printed in China

Contents

THE FIVE-MINUTE APPROACH

LOOKING AFTER YOUR HANDS

We all aspire to elegant, perfectly manicured hands, usually with long, polished nails. Unfortunately, long nails are not always practical. Even though the advertisements tell us that we should possess perfect nails that never crack, chip or break, such routine activities as opening drawers and dialing telephones can be devastating to them. Of course, the models in the nail advertisements do nothing more arduous than caressing polish bottles – their nails are not constantly endangered by doing the laundry or washing their hair. Even if you are fortunate enough to possess good, healthy nails, the struggle to maintain a uniform set of ten is a tough one. Although there is no magic formula for beautiful nails, there are a lot of things you can do to help maintain them, and none of them will add more than five minutes to your beauty routine.

Manicuring may seem like a mysterious art, only to be practiced by professionals with vast trays of special equipment. It is actually quite simple, once you understand how nails actually "work". The part of the nail that we can see (the nail plate) is made up of layers of dead protein, attached to the nail bed beneath it (see diagram). These protein layers do contain some oil and moisture, but they need to be kept flexible and supple in order to prevent them from breaking. Nails start growing from the matrix, which is underneath the base of the nail, and sometimes a patch of this live nail can be seen. It is called the lanula, or "half-moon". The cuticle, which protects the base of the nail and seals the matrix off from any bacteria which might otherwise work their way beneath the skin, extends around the base and sides of the nail plate.

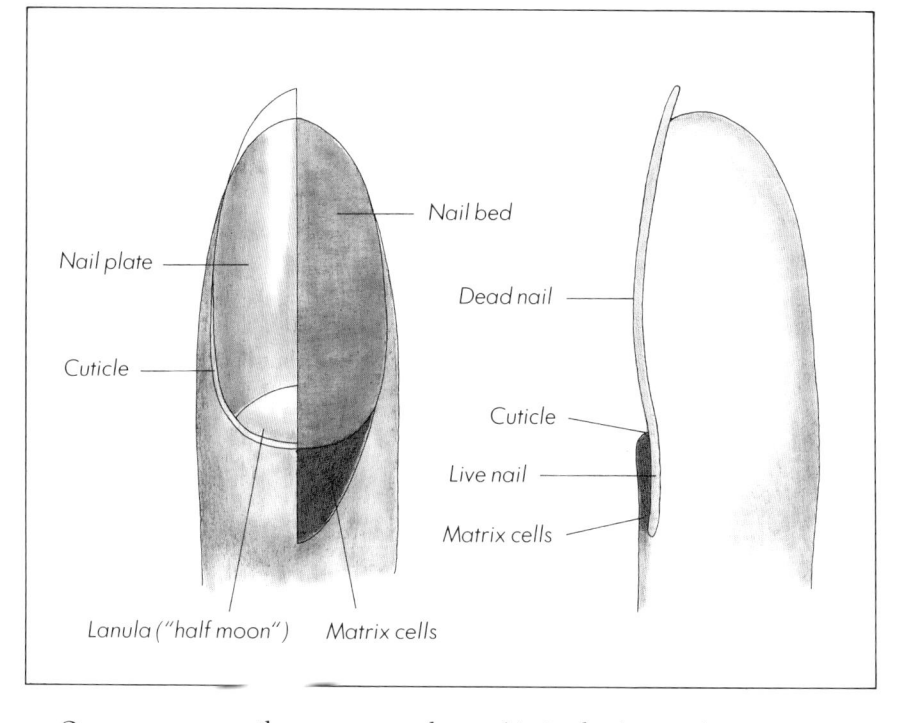

Nail bed

Nail plate

Cuticle

Dead nail

Cuticle

Live nail

Matrix cells

Lanula ("half moon")   Matrix cells

On average, nails grow at about ⅛ inch (4 mm) per month. Of course growth varies from person to person, and, generally speaking, young people's nails grow faster than old people's. Nail growth is stimulated during pregnancy, and in the spring and summer months.

Illness or emotional stress may slow down or even stop nail growth. Signs of ill-health and internal disorders can manifest themselves in nails in the form of splitting, flaking, white specks and ridges or furrows. Cases of anemia, for example, can be diagnosed from a characteristic colorlessness, or an overly curved "spoon" shape to the nails. A well-balanced diet with plenty of vitamins and minerals is just as important for nails as it is for any other part of your body.

PRACTICAL TIPS

- Over frequent applications of polish and the consequent use of polish remover can make your nails brittle or fragile. Most nail polish remover contains acetone, which makes nails very dry. If you can track down a remover which does not contain it, so much the better.

- Detergent is another culprit, so always wear rubber gloves when washing dishes. In fact, it is a good idea to wear them for most household chores, because the chemicals contained in cleaning materials won't do your nails any good, either.

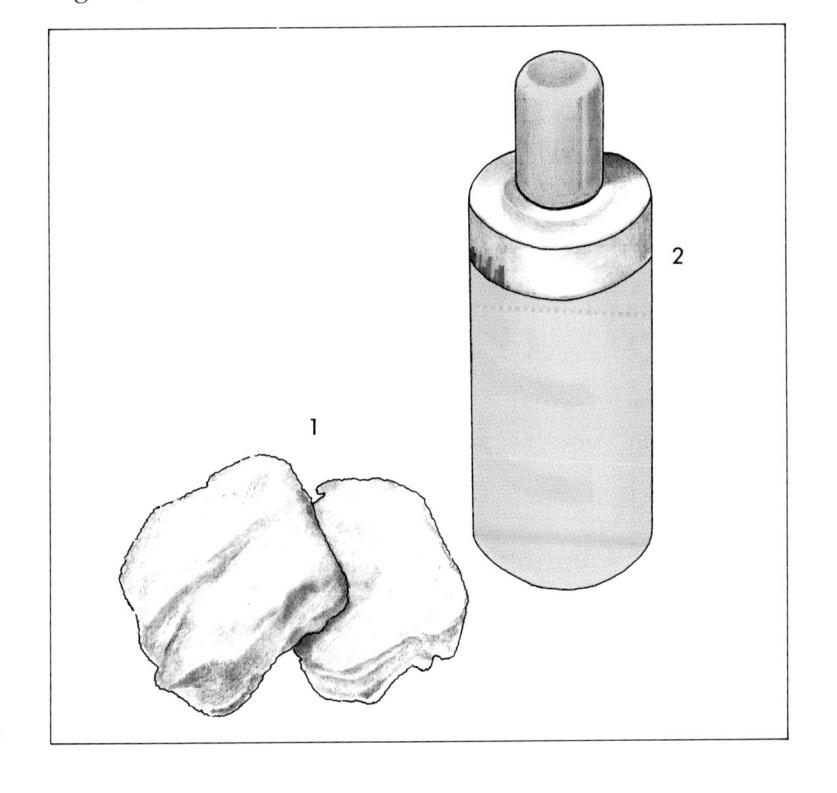

1 Cotton pads
2 Nail polish remover

- If you work in the garden, make sure you have a pair of gloves for outdoor work. For gardening jobs where gloves are not practical, apply a layer of hand cream, and work some soap under your fingernails before you start. This will save you from having to poke out particles of ingrained soil later.

- If your hands are covered in oil and grease, apply a special heavy-duty hand cleanser designed for this purpose before washing them. This is far better than painfully scrubbing away with a harsh, bristled brush and a bar of soap.

- The best way to apply hand cream is to smooth it on over each finger, as if you were sliding on a ring. For the palm and back of your hand, work the cream into the skin with circular massaging movements of your thumb and fingers. If your nails are very dry and flaky, apply a little moisturizer to them whenever you are using it on your face or body, and keep a pot of hand cream by the sink for use after washing your hands.

- There are several exfoliants available that help to get rid of any dry skin from your hands. If you have a few extra minutes, this is a good way to start your basic manicure. An exfoliant also comes in handy for use on feet and elbows. Remember to moisturize afterwards.

- If your fingers are discolored or stained with nicotine, rub the skin with the cut half of a lemon. Lemon juice contains a useful natural bleaching agent which can also be helpful in removing freckles. If you should find yourself acquiring "age" or "liver" spots on the backs of your hands, you can soak them in lemon juice mixed with oil once a week. This will not remove them entirely, but you will find that it helps to minimize them.

1 *Massage oil*
2 *Hand towel*

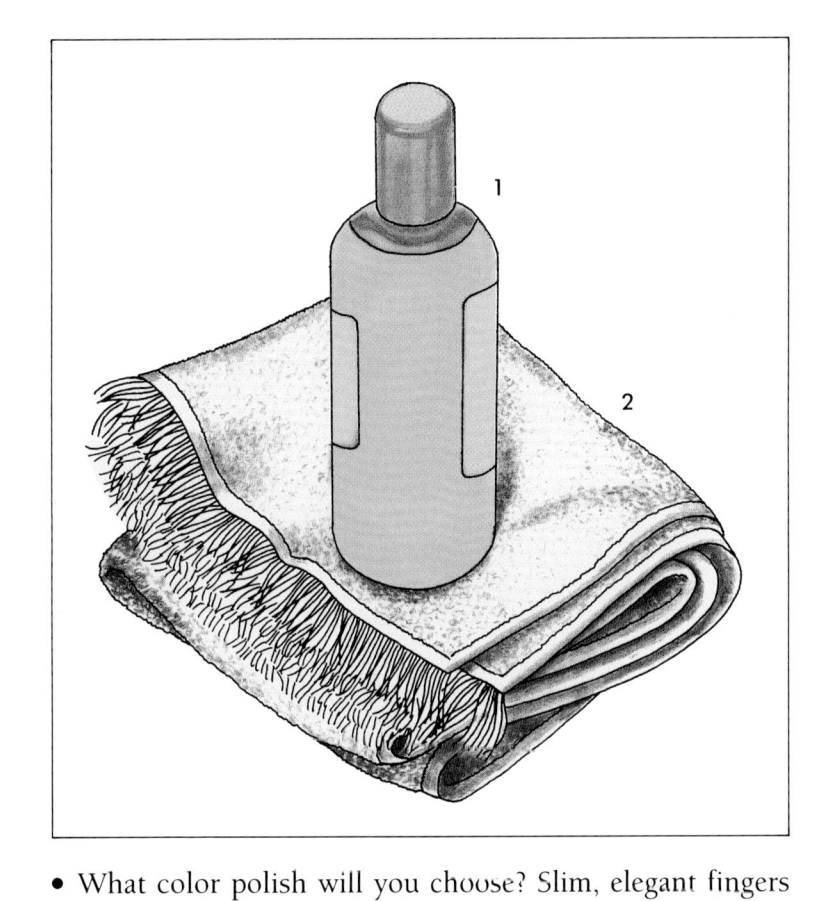

- What color polish will you choose? Slim, elegant fingers look good with any shade. However, if your hands are not your most attractive feature, avoid using bright colors that will draw attention to them; stick to the more natural-looking colors.

- Nails can become stained by the pigment in a dark-colored polish. Usually, the application of a base coat under the color will prevent this pigment from marking your nail. However, should this happen, it is probably best left to go away of its own accord. There are bleaches, but they contain hydrogen peroxide, which has a very drying effect on nails.

- To remove nail polish effectively, moisten a cotton ball with remover, and wrap it around your nail, pressing it firmly for a few seconds to help dissolve the polish before wiping it clean. Use a fresh cotton ball for each nail and, to avoid smearing your fingers with polish, work through your nails methodically, from your thumb to your little finger, finishing one hand before you begin the other. If you are using an acetone remover, massage in a little cuticle oil before applying new polish.

- Finally, remember that however much you manicure and moisturize, the best maintained set of nails will quickly disintegrate if you abuse them. Don't use them as tools. They are not a kit for scraping off labels and prising off lids, so contain your impatience until you find something designed for the job you want to do – it will be worth it in the end!

LOOKING AFTER YOUR FEET
Ever since Cinderella's ugly sisters chopped off their toes to fit the glass slipper, generations of women have endured discomfort in shoes. Fashionable, attractive footwear always seems to have some drawback – toes too pointed, heels too high, not enough support for the foot, or, in the case of mules, the sheer effort of keeping them on one's feet. The majority of problems women have with their feet are caused by ill-fitting shoes, so footwear should be chosen carefully. High heels are fine – but you don't have to wear them every-day. Vary your shoes and, most important, your heel height from day to day. When you are selecting a pair of shoes from your closet, consider what you might be doing during the

day. If it's a lot of walking, very high heels are obviously not appropriate, and will make your feet painful and tired. You should never buy a pair of shoes which feel as if they are going to need a lot of 'breaking in'; a good pair of new shoes should be flexible and comfortable.

PRACTICAL TIPS

- It is a good idea to kick your shoes off whenever you get the chance. Wiggle your toes, rotate your ankles and give your feet a shake. Another useful exercise is placing a ball under your foot and moving it around (see pages 72 and 74 for further foot and ankle exercises).

- Relax and literally 'put your feet up' if you have been standing for long periods of time, as this will help to prevent varicose veins. Unfortunately, these tend to run in families – however, anything that restricts the blood flow to the legs or increases the pressure on them should be avoided. Exercise is beneficial, as is a diet containing plenty of fiber.

- It is wonderful to be able to kick your shoes off and walk barefoot, but stick to grass and mud. Don't go barefoot on hard surfaces like asphalt for long distances.

- Your feet, like every other part of your body, need regular moisturizing. Dry cracked skin on the feet can be painful, and a regular application of moisturizer or body lotion will make all the difference. If any area is especially dry, a heavy-duty lanolin-based cream can be obtained at most drugstores. If deep fissures have formed in your heels, you should make an appointment with a chiropodist. In order to prevent these forming, tackle hard skin regularly – but not too roughly – with a pumice stone or a rough skin remover.

- Chilblains on both hands and feet are encouraged by changes of temperature, so don't expose them to the cold and then go straight indoors and cuddle a radiator. Make sure your footwear is dry, and try to keep your feet warm in winter – but don't roast them in front of the fire as this may cause chapped skin.

PRODUCTS AND EQUIPMENT

Artificial Nails: These are very useful as emergency measures when a nail is broken. A full set of artificial nails can look wonderful, but it needs a great deal of maintenance. Acrylic nails are also available, but they are very difficult to apply and should be done by a trained manicurist.

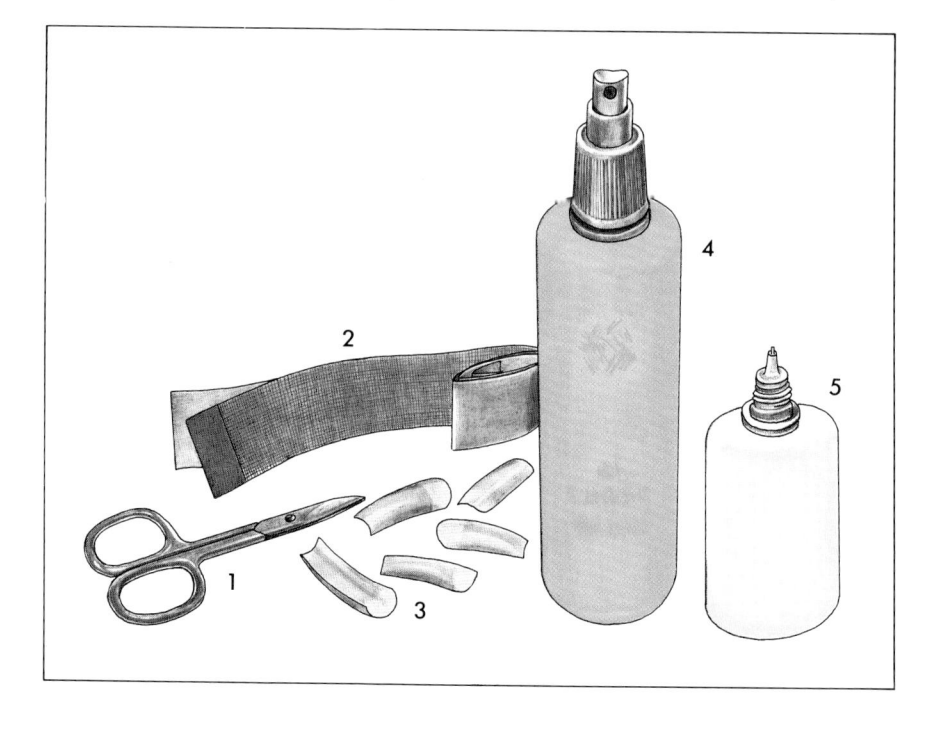

1 *Nail scissors*
2 *Nail wrap*
3 *Artificial nails*
4 *Activator spray*
5 *Glue*

1 Nail buffer
2 Orange stick
3 Hoof stick
4 Cuticle clippers
5 Nail treatment oil
6 Nail polish
7 Base coat
8 Top coat
9 Cuticle cream
10 Quick-dry spray
11 Nail bath
12 Emery boards
13 Nail scissors

Base coat: A coat of this applied under your polish is useful because it not only protects your nail, it also helps to prevent the polish from chipping by acting as an added adhesive between it and your nail plate.

Buffer: These come in all shapes and sizes. The most practical is a three-way buffer, which combines three different buffing surfaces, so that you can really build up a shine. There are also the larger, more old-fashioned buffers, which are traditionally used in conjunction with a dab of paste polish. These usually have a polishing cloth which may be taken off and washed, so they tend to be longer lasting.

Cuticle cream: This cream, for softening and nourishing cuticles, can be used on both fingernails and toenails. Most brands contain lanolin and petroleum jelly. Cuticle oils, for keeping the skin around the nail soft, are also available.

Cuticle clippers: Similar to nail clippers, these are useful for cutting back cuticles and dealing with hangnails.

Foot bath: Although these can be bought, a plastic bowl of warm soapy water (moisturizing liquid soap) will be just as relaxing.

Glue (resin) and activator spray (fixative): A tube of glue is a handy item in any manicure kit. It is best to get a little set of spray, glue with a detachable nozzle, and a glue remover. The activator spray, or fixative, should be used in conjunction with the glue when fitting fiberglass nail wraps (below). Hold it at least 6 inches (15.5 cms) away from your hand when spraying and be careful not to get any in your eyes.

Hand mask: Essentially the same as a face mask, applied to the hands.

Nail clippers: Both fingernail and toenail clippers are available from most drugstores. For toenails, clippers are preferable to scissors.

Nail file: Emery boards are the best type of nail file, and they come in various weights. Very coarse emery boards and steel files are best avoided. Larger, heavy variants are available for the feet, to smooth down calluses and rough skin. (The alternative, rubbing heels with a pumice stone in the bath, is equally effective.)

Nail Polish (or Enamel): Polish will certainly help to protect your nails, but claims that it will actually nourish them are dubious. It is used to best advantage in conjunction with

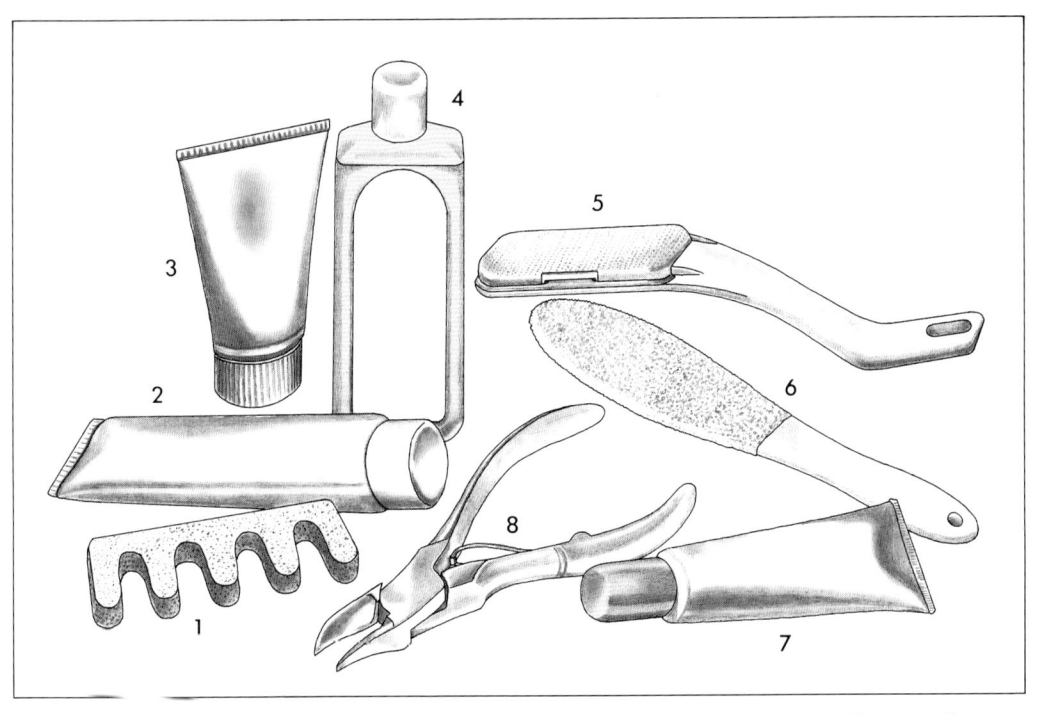

1 Toenail separators
2 Exfoliant
3 Sunscreen
4 Body lotion
5 Metal foot file
6 Plastic foot file
7 Handmask
8 Toenail clippers

a base coat and top coat. You should always allow sufficient time for two coats of polish to dry. Both liquid and aerosol 'quick-dry' products for nails are available, but they are of limited use and tend to make the polish lose its sheen.

Nail Polish Remover: These contain organic solvents such as acetone for dissolving old polish.

Nail Strengthener: Used to help prevent fragile nails from splitting or tearing, strengtheners can be applied to the nail before the base coat.

Nail Wraps: Made from silk, linen or fiberglass, these are a comparatively new addition to the manicure kit, and are available in sheets which can be cut to size.

Orange sticks and hoof sticks: Both are useful for pushing back cuticles, although a hoof stick with a rubber-tipped end is best. If you are using an orange stick, wrap a little cotton around the end to soften it.

Ridge filler: If your nails have a slightly grooved surface, this can be applied under a base coat to smooth them.

Top coat: This should be applied over dry nail polish. Like the base coat, it protects the polish by acting as a sealant.

SOME PROBLEMS

Athlete's Foot: This is a fungal infection, most commonly found between the toes. It can be treated with surgical spirit to dry out the skin, and anti-fungal creams. To prevent it, dry thoroughly between the toes after washing.

Bunions: An enlarging of the toe joint, usually on the big toe. Often very painful, the most common cause of bunions is ill-fitting, tight shoes. Once bunions have developed, there is little that can be done apart from wearing comfortable shoes and padding them to ease the pressure on the bunion. Surgery, a last resort, is often unsatisfactory.

Corns: These develop as a result of pressure or friction, usually on the toes. Medicated corn pads and removers are available at drugstores, but if corns persist, they should be treated by a chiropodist.

Foot odour: If this is a problem, you can help to prevent it by wearing natural fibers next to your skin. After bathing, apply surgical spirit foot spray or talcum powder.

Hangnails: Pieces of skin torn away from, but still attached to, the base or side of a fingernail. These are caused by the cuticle splitting around the nail, often as a result of incorrect cuticle removal. They can usually be taken care of with a cuticle clipper, but if you are concerned about them go to a professional manicurist.

Ingrown Toenails: Incorrect trimming and filing, or an injury to the toe, can cause the edge of the nail to grow into the skin. These can be very painful and should be treated by a doctor.

Leuconychia (white spots): These are either caused by general wear and tear, or by blows to the matrix of the nail. They have also been linked to a zinc deficiency, so try to ensure that you have enough in your diet (seafood is a rich source). They will grow out naturally, with the nail.

Nail Biting: There are a number of ways to kick this habit – try painting them with one of the special foul-tasting solutions from the drugstore, or with neat bitter aloes which is even more unpleasant. If all else fails, you could try applying artificial nails, as even the most hardened nail biter will have difficulty chewing through them.

Paraonychia: Inflammation of the skin surrounding the nail, often caused by a bacterial infection. Wearing rubber gloves for any wet job can go a long way to prevent this, but if it occurs you should see a doctor.

Verruca: A highly contagious viral wart-like infection found on the sole of the foot. It is usually easy to get rid of, either by seeking advice from your doctor or chiropodist, or using home remedies from the drugstore.

Warts: These are often found on the hands, but they can occur on any part of the body. Usually dark in color with a rough, horny surface, many, if left untreated, will eventually disappear of their own accord. If you feel that they are unsightly, see your doctor about having them removed.

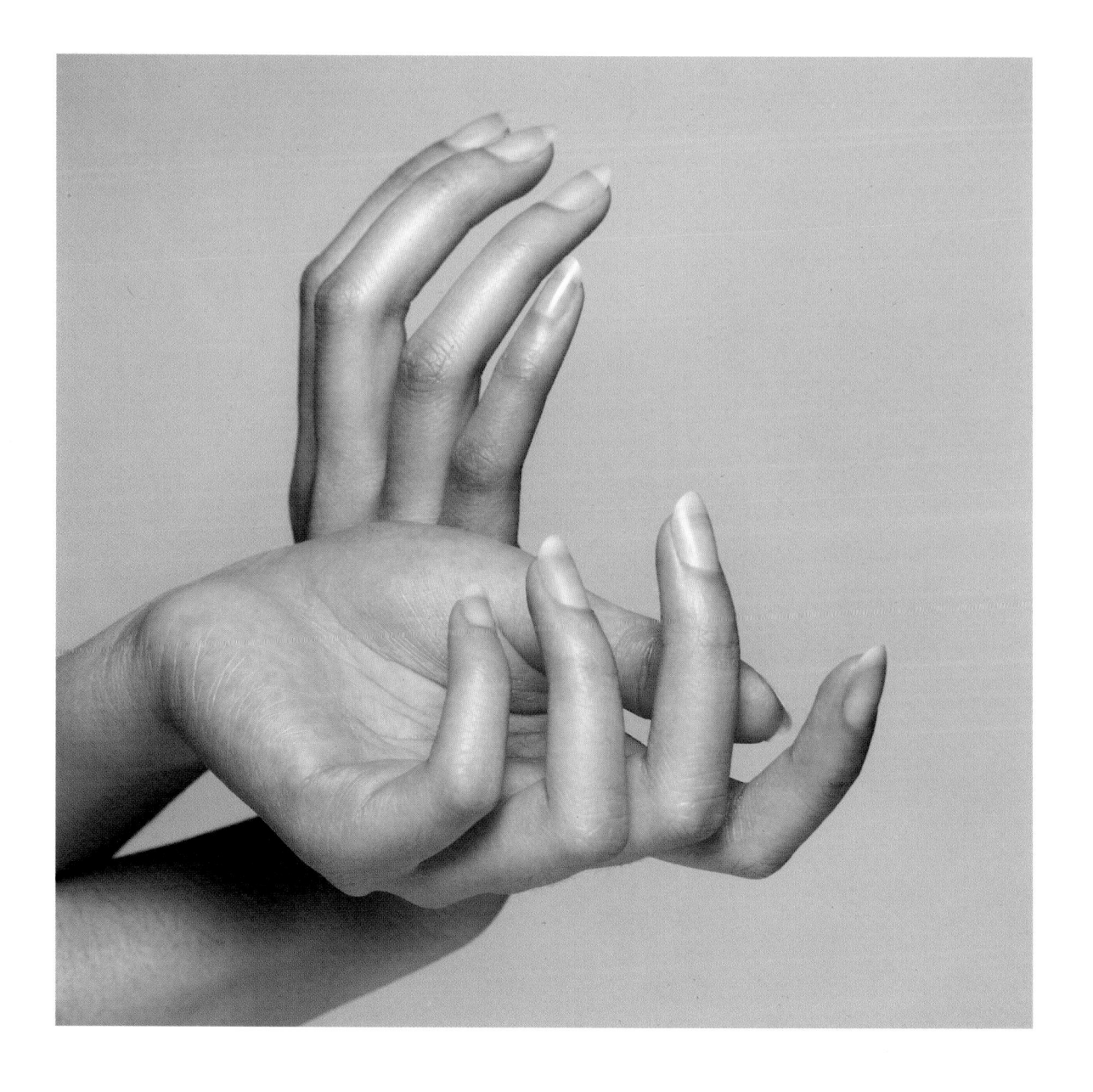

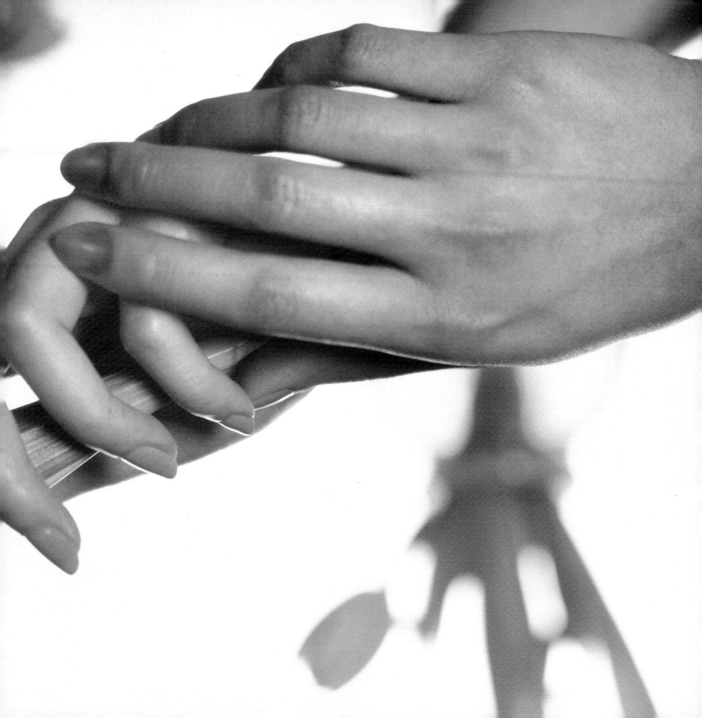

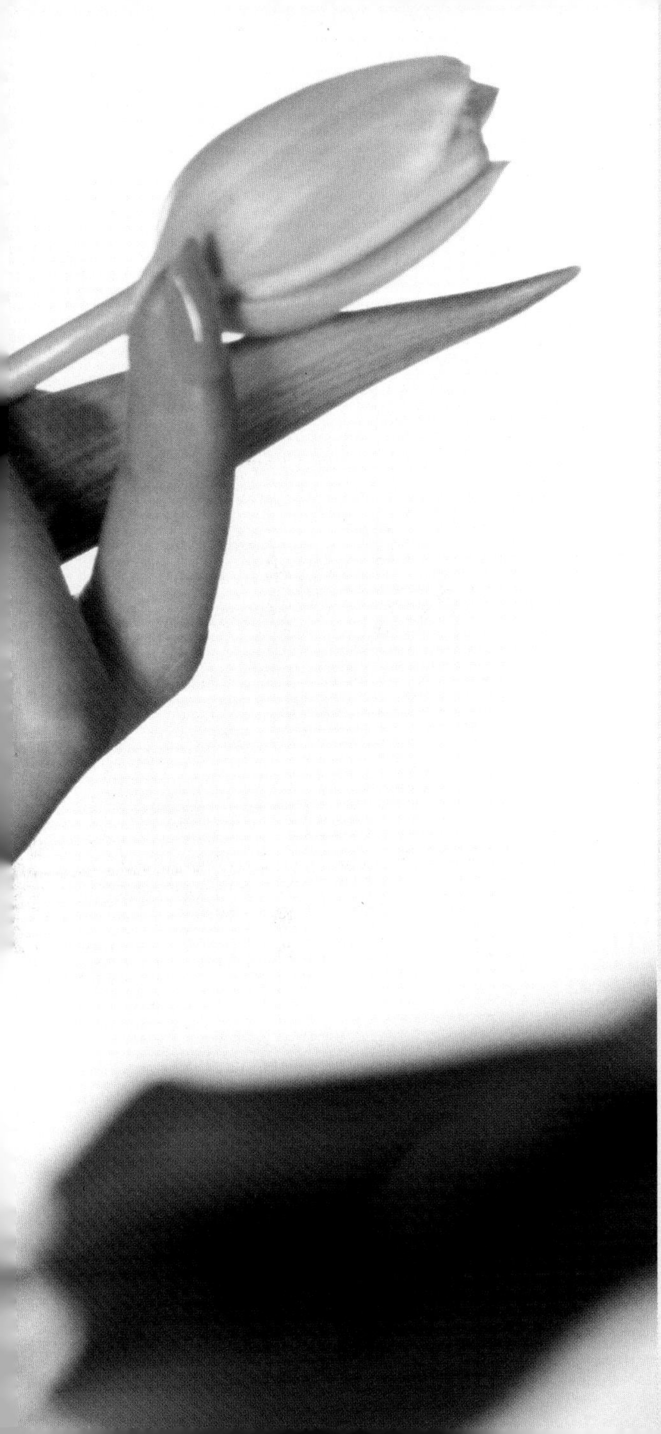

1
MANICURES

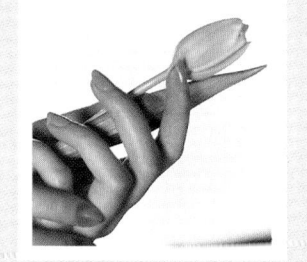

CUTICLE CARE

What you need
Cuticle cream
Hoof stick or orange
   stick
Bowl of warm soapy
   water
Cuticle clippers
Towel

Cuticles are important because they protect the base of all the vital matrix cells (see page 7). So, although it may seem like a time-saver, resist the temptation to poke your cuticles back with the nearest sharp object, or you may end up with sore, red-rimmed nails. You may also damage the lanula or 'half-moon' at the base of the nail and so affect the new nail growth. To keep your cuticles neat, and help prevent hangnails, push them back gently with the towel when you dry your hands. For manicuring, use either a rubber-ended hoof stick or an orange stick with its tip wrapped in cotton.

Cuticle cream is used to soften the cuticle. A cuticle oil, usually containing almond oil, can also be used, or, if your drugstore does not stock it, try baby oil. Massage it well into your cuticles and the skin surrounding them with the ball of your thumb. This helps to stimulate your circulation, giving your nails an attractive pink glow.

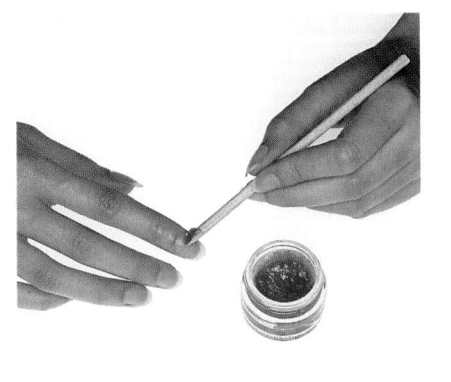

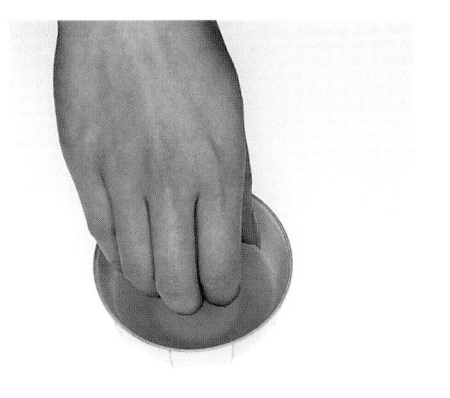

1 *Apply a small amount of cuticle cream to each cuticle with a hoof stick. Massage it in with circular motions of the thumb.*

2 *Soak fingertips in a bowl of warm soapy water for at least one minute. Dry thoroughly afterwards.*

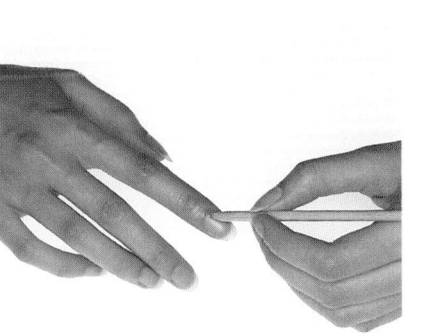

3 *Push back cuticles very gently with a hoof stick.*

4 *Trim any hangnails carefully with cuticle clippers.*

TRIMMING YOUR NAILS

What you need
Nail scissors
Nail file

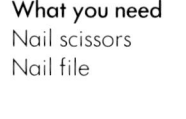

Although long fingernails look very glamorous, short nails can look fabulous, too, if they are clean and well-kept. There may be times when it is more appropriate to keep your nails trimmed – if, for example, you are a keen gardener or do a lot of cooking – and less healthy nails will certainly look better if they are kept short. Cutting your nails is not the ideal way of shortening them, but if you want to take off a length of nail, it is much quicker than filing.

Choose scissors in preference to clippers, as these can cause cracks.

Always remove polish before cutting your nails. As with filing (see page 26), you can make one single cut straight across the top of your nail if you prefer a squared-off finish to a rounded one. Otherwise, nails should be cut on each side, going from the edge to the center. When you are cutting your nails, concentrate on the length you want, rather than the shape. This can be achieved afterwards, with a file.

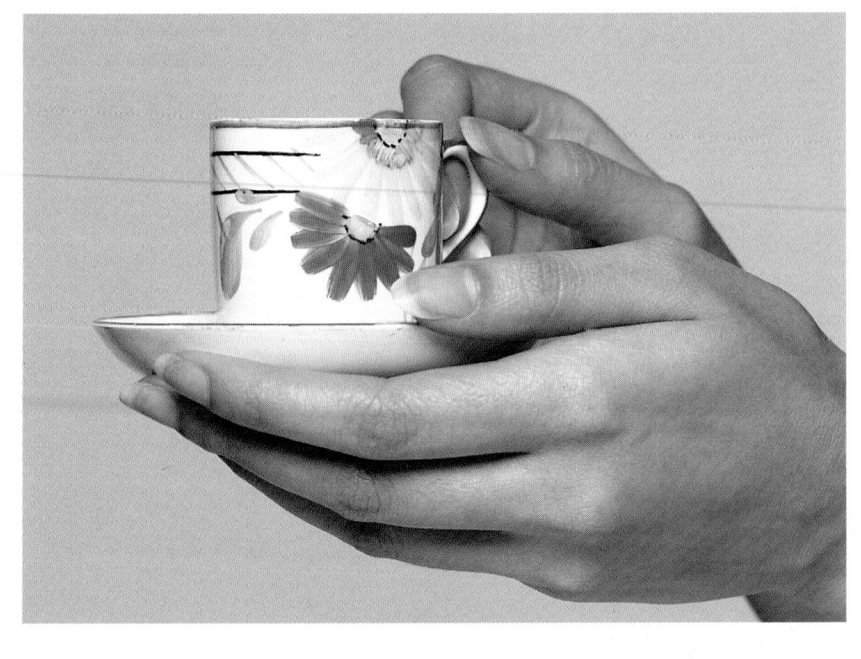

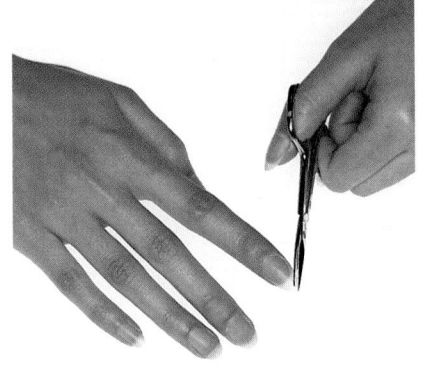

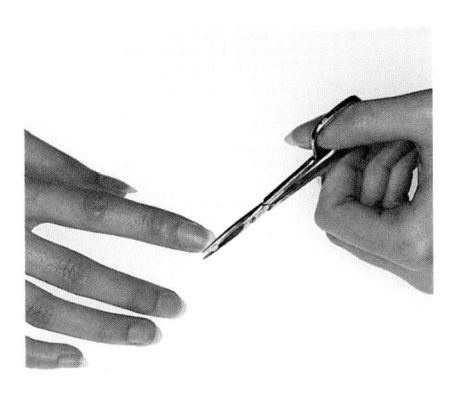

1 *Cut from the side to the middle of the nail, to the desired length.*

2 *Repeat on the other side. Don't worry about the final shape at this point.*

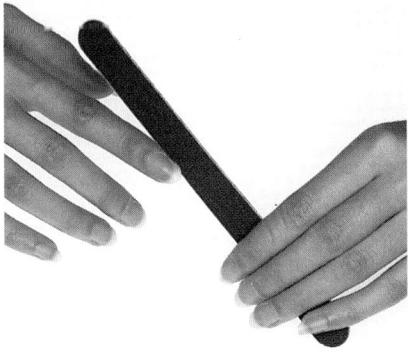

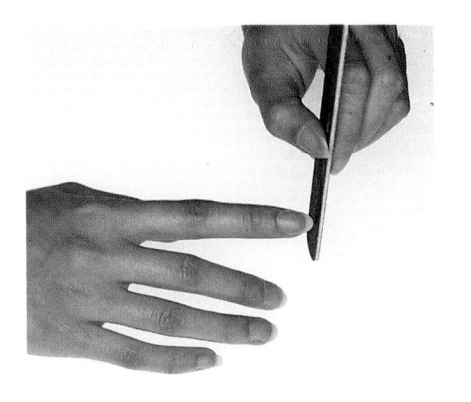

3 *File each side of your nail from the sides to the center, holding the file at an angle of 45° (see page 26).*

4 *Holding the file vertically, file the tip of the nail using a downward motion.*

FILING YOUR NAILS

What you need
Nail file

Generally speaking, it is better to file your nails than to cut them. Steel files may last a long time, but, because they are harsh and inflexible, they can tear or split your nails. Buy a packet of fine emery boards instead.

Before you start, decide which shape will suit your nails best. Square nails, unless they are very long, give your hands a practical look, which may not always be flattering if your fingers are short. Although easier to break, rounded nails tend to look more elegant.

For rounded nails, always file from the edge to the middle, trying to achieve a nice smooth curve. Never file back and forth, as this can cause the nail layers to split, and be careful not to file right down into the corners, as this can cause ingrown nails.

Most importantly, your nails should all be the same length – it is not worth hanging onto that one long nail in the hope that the others will eventually catch up with it.

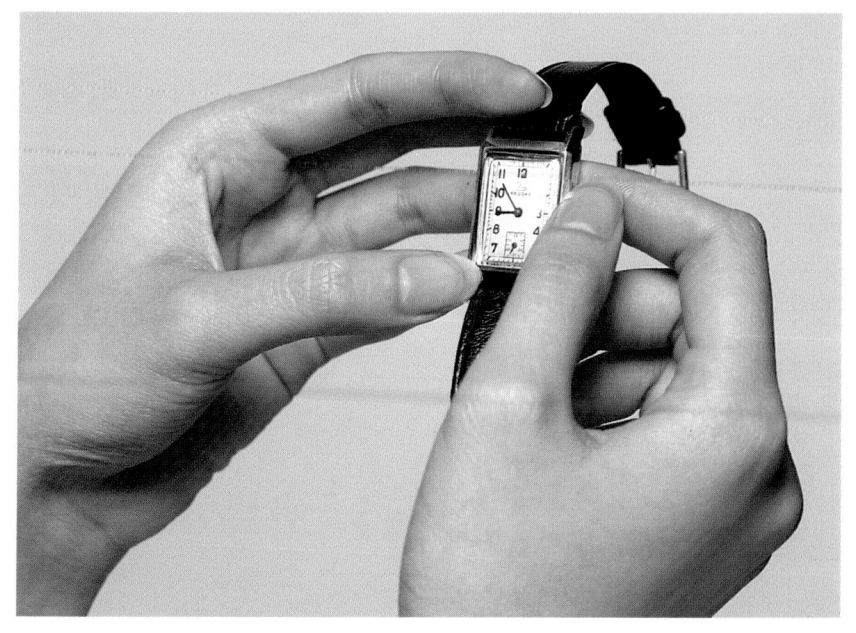

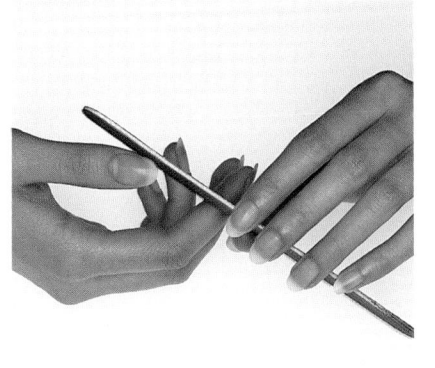

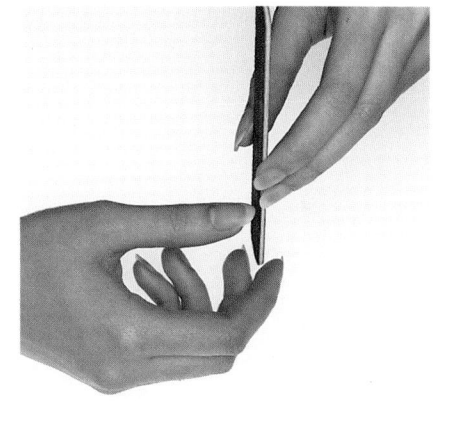

Round   **1** *File each side of your nail from the side to the center, holding the emery board at an angle of 45°.*

2 *Holding the file vertically, file the tip of the nail using a downward motion.*

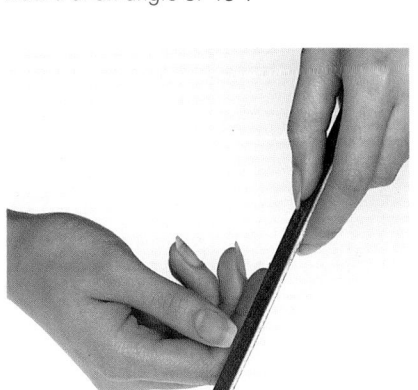

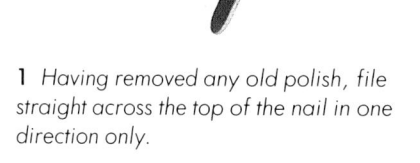

Square   **1** *Having removed any old polish, file straight across the top of the nail in one direction only.*

2 *Holding the file vertically, file the tip of the nail using a downward motion.*

INSTANT NAIL REPAIRS

What you need
Glue
Nail file
Nail strengthener

A single tear in a perfect set of nails can be heartbreaking, especially if you have worked hard to get them in good condition. However, if you act quickly, it may be possible to repair the nail with glue. Assess the tear to see if it is worth saving, but don't fiddle with it. Remove any polish from the nail beforehand, since polish that has been stuck down with glue is impossible to get rid of with an ordinary polish remover, and has to be whittled away with a file.

Nail glue is available from most drugstores – it is a useful thing to have in your nail kit at all times. If possible, buy a brand of glue which comes with a nozzle, as it is very easy to overdo it – and very frustrating when your fingers get stuck together. Once the glue is safely on your nail, make sure that it is hardened before you buff. Once you have completed the buffing and applied a couple of coats of nail strengthener, the tear should hardly be visible.

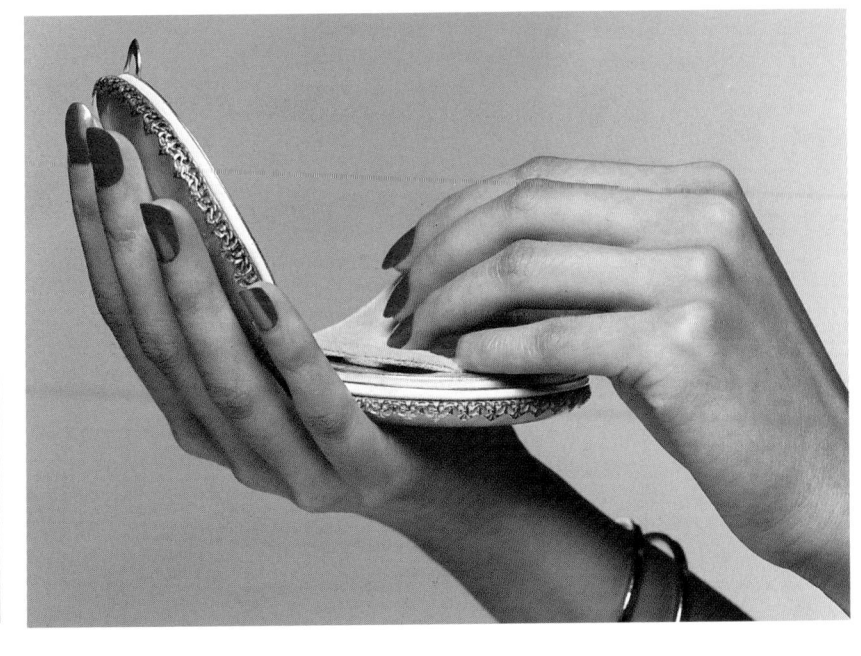

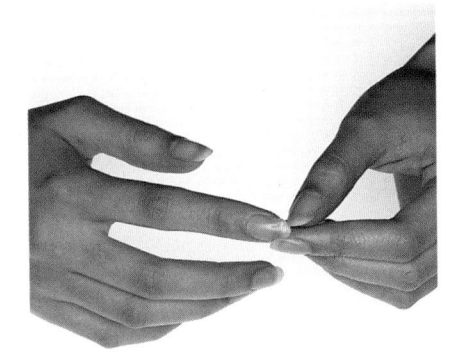

1 *Apply glue sparingly along the line of the break.*

2 *Hold the edges of the nail together while the glue sets.*

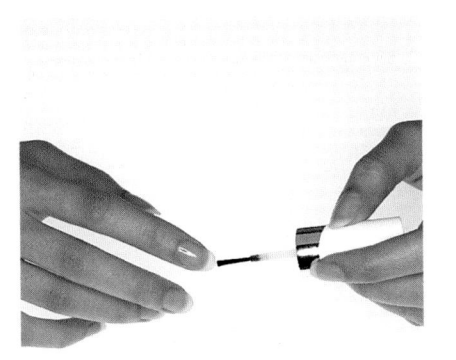

3 *Buff the repaired area, and paint whole nail with strengthener.*

Buff up and clear polish

What you need
Nail buffer
Cuticle oil
Nail polish remover
Cotton ball
Clear polish

Healthy, shining nails are the best finishing touch for a natural looking make-up. Practical and versatile, they will go with every outfit in your closet, from a sweat suit to a cocktail dress.

Buffing won't dry out your nails at all and is an excellent way of stimulating the circulation and smoothing the nail surface. If your nails are in a poor condition, it is far better to treat them to a good buffing than to try and disguise them by slapping on coats of polish.

We have used a liquid polish here, but if you prefer it, paste polish may be used instead. Apply a small amount of the paste to each nail with an orange stick, and buff with firm downward strokes from the base of the nail to the edge, lifting the buffer after each stroke.

Here, we show a three-way buffer, which is much handier than the large, old-fashioned type. You should work through all three sections, from the roughest to the very smoothest.

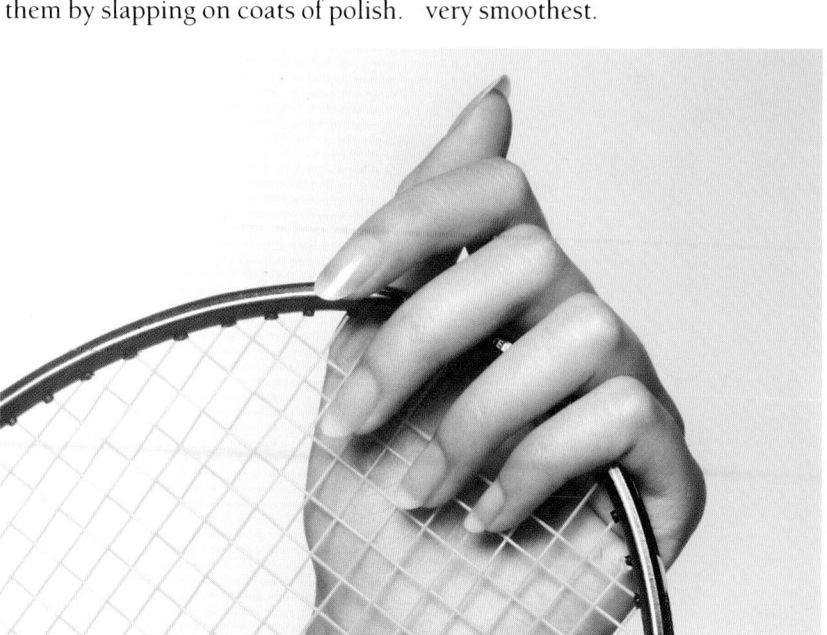

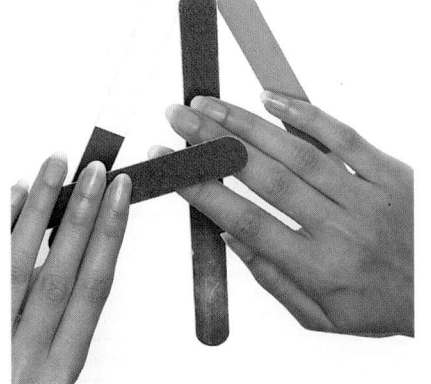

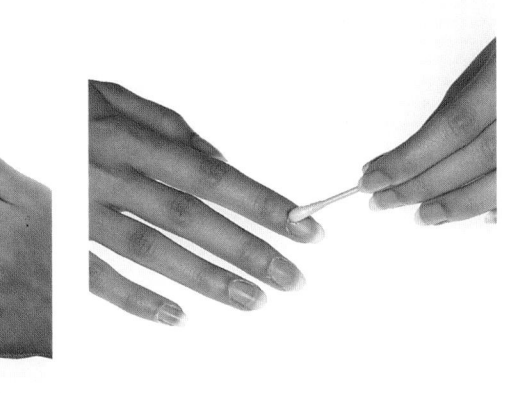

1 *Buff your nails, using all the sections of a three-way buffer.*

2 *Apply oil around cuticle to remove any dust created by buffing. Massage it in with the ball of your thumb.*

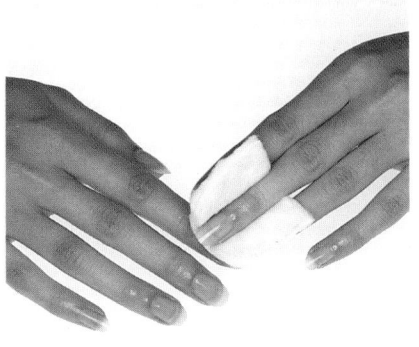

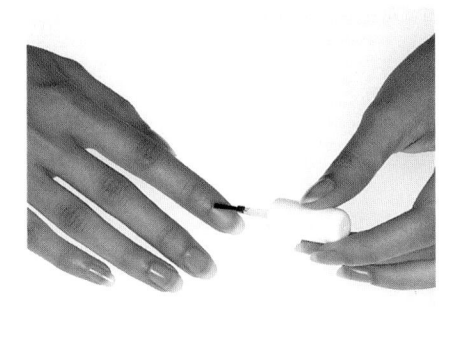

3 *Remove oil with a touch of nail polish remover and wipe dry with cotton ball.*

4 *Apply clear liquid polish. If you are using paste polish, buff your nails after applying.*

Painting your nails

What you need
Base coat
Colored nail polish

Beautifully colored nails give any outfit a chic, finished look, and this deep red will go equally well with a tailored suit or a cocktail dress.

For a strong color, you should apply two coats of polish, always over a transparent base coat. Apply the first coat sparingly, but don't worry about allowing the polish to dry between coats: the first nail will be dry enough for a re-application by the time you get back to it. Try to leave a hair space between the polish and your cuticles, so that it doesn't spill over onto your fingers.

Paint each nail with three strokes only: the first straight down the middle, followed by one stroke on either side. If the polish smudges, dip an orange stick in some remover and carefully wipe it away.

Ideally, you should allow your nails about half an hour to be completely dry. There's a world of difference between 'touch-dry' and hard, and there are few things more irritating then a smudge on an otherwise perfect set of nails.

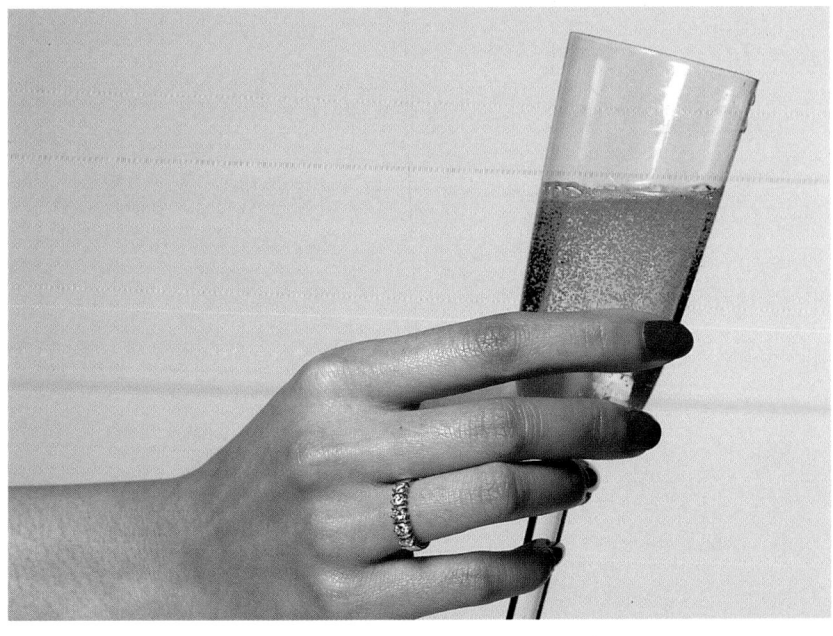

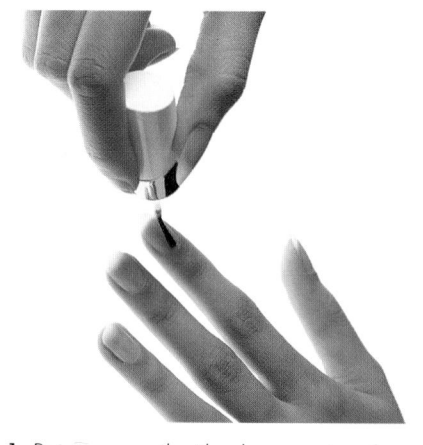

1 *Paint your nail with a base coat so the polish is less likely to chip.*

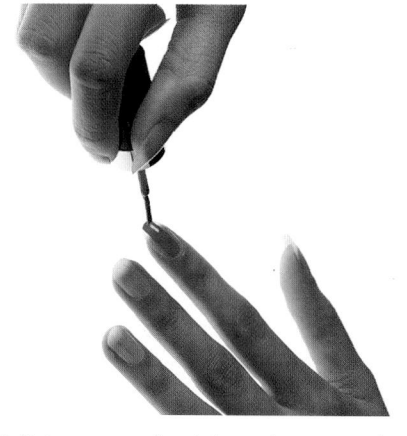

2 *Paint a strip of red down the center of your nail.*

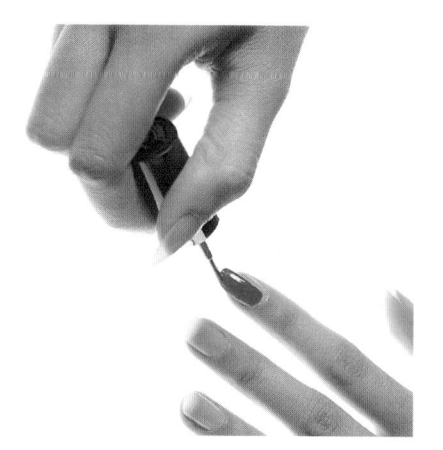

3 *Paint down the sides – a single stroke for each.*

REPAIRING CHIPPED POLISH

What you need
Nail buffer
Nail polish

Nail polish chips for a number of reasons: either the polish has been applied too thickly or without a base coat or top coat, the nail is in a dry and flaky condition, or there is oil or moisture on the nail surface. But the most expertly applied polish will, after a couple of days, become chipped from general wear and tear and need repairing.

It is usually best to try and repair chipped polish, rather than getting out the remover, because you may end up unwittingly removing polish from other nails. However, if the rest of the polish on the chipped nail is flaking away, then it may be best to remove it, and start again.

When you are painting over the chipped area, just "dab" it lightly with the brush. (Always paint your nails in strips from the base to the end of the nail, never from side to side.) If you are in a tearing hurry, you can apply a quick-drying spray or a gentle blast of warm air from your hairdryer, but don't hold it too close to your nails.

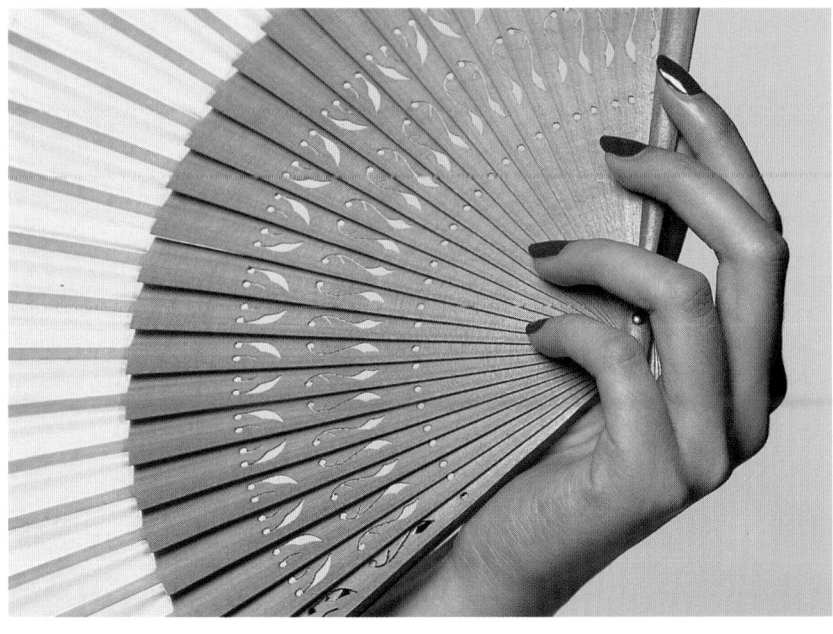

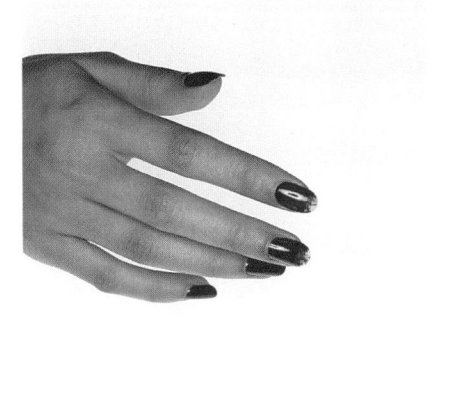

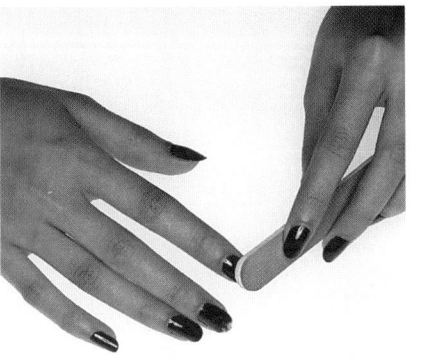

1 *Take a close look at the chipped area, to see if it is worth repairing.*

2 *Using a medium weight buffer, smooth over the chipped area.*

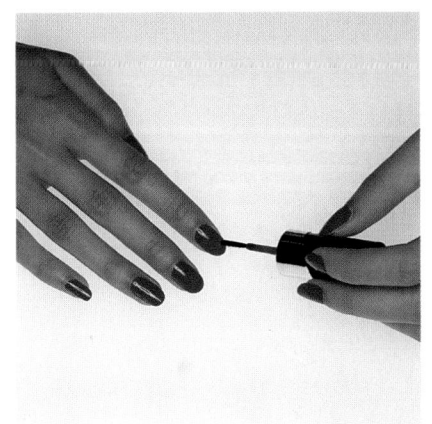

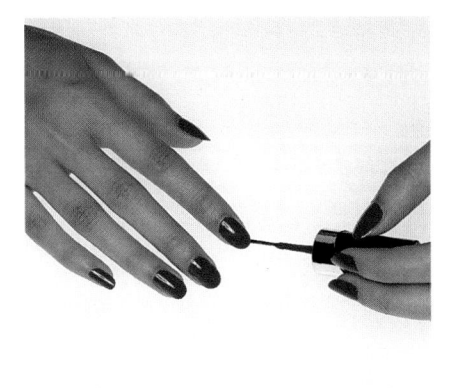

3 *Paint over the chipped area with a thin layer of polish.*

4 *Wait until this is 'touch-dry', and then paint over the entire nail.*

FRENCH MANICURE

What you need
Base coat
White nail polish
Pale pink nail polish
Top coat

This chic variation on the natural look has become very popular, and is very useful if you have a number of quick changes to perform and no time for taking off and re-applying colored polish. Until recently, it was necessary to color underneath your nail tip with a white pencil to achieve this look, but now there are complete French manicure kits available, containing a base coat, a white polish to be painted across the nail tips, a natural looking pink polish, and a top coat.

French manicures look especially good if you have a white 'half moon' or lanula showing at the base of your nail, but if you can't see them all, don't try to force your cuticles back as you may damage the living nail underneath.

It is important to wait until the white polish on the nail tips is *thoroughly* dry before applying the pink over it. With a base coat and a top coat, a single application of the pink polish will be sufficient, as it should not be completely opaque.

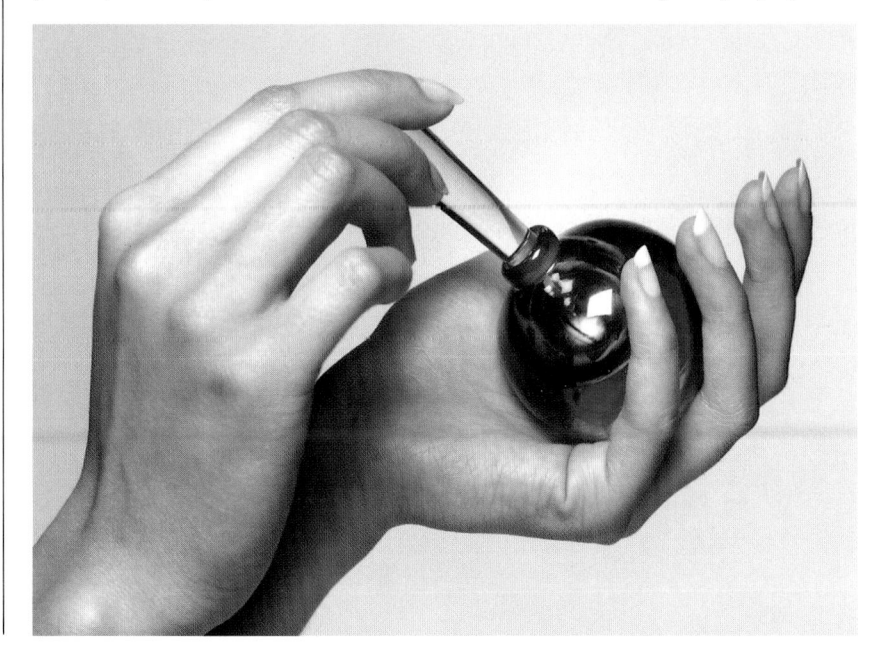

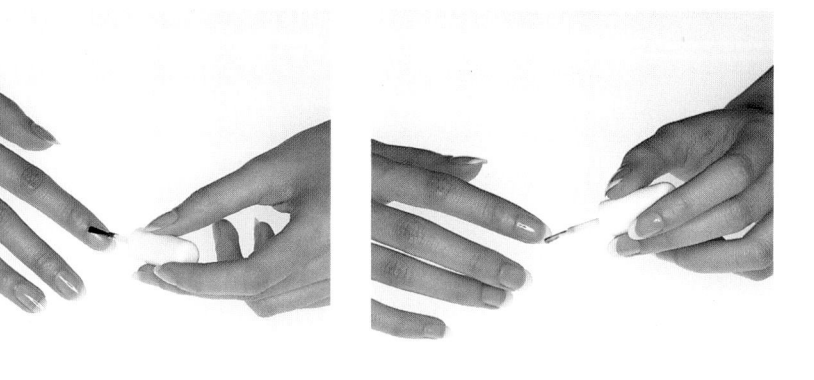

1 *Apply base coat to protect your nails and help prevent chipping.*

2 *Apply two thin coats of white polish to the nail tips in a single stroke from side to side.*

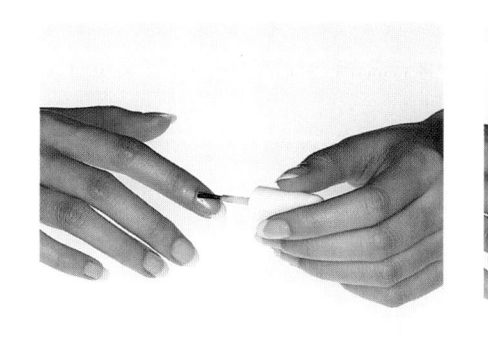

3 *Once the white polish is completely dry, apply pink polish over entire nail.*

4 *Apply top coat over entire nail, for extra protection.*

Nail wrapping

What you need
Nail buffer
Nail scissors
Nail wrap
Glue
Activator spray

If you are tired of finding your nails breaking just as you have succeeded in growing them to a reasonable length, you could try using nail wraps. "Wrapping" your nails with prepared strips of silk, linen or fiberglass is an excellent method of strengthening them. Like artificial nails, the wraps will "grow" with your real nail, and the gap that is left at the base will need filling periodically with a small strip of fiberglass. This may, in the long run, prove considerably more time-consuming than a regular manicure routine, but the pay-off will be the absence of broken, cracked or torn nails.

Make sure that the wrap is placed in position on your nail before applying any glue to it. The glue will soak through the wrap, making it adhere to your nail. It should be perfectly dry before you begin buffing.

Make sure that you cut the wrap to the exact shape of your nail – if you use the glue carefully, you can trim the end once it is in place.

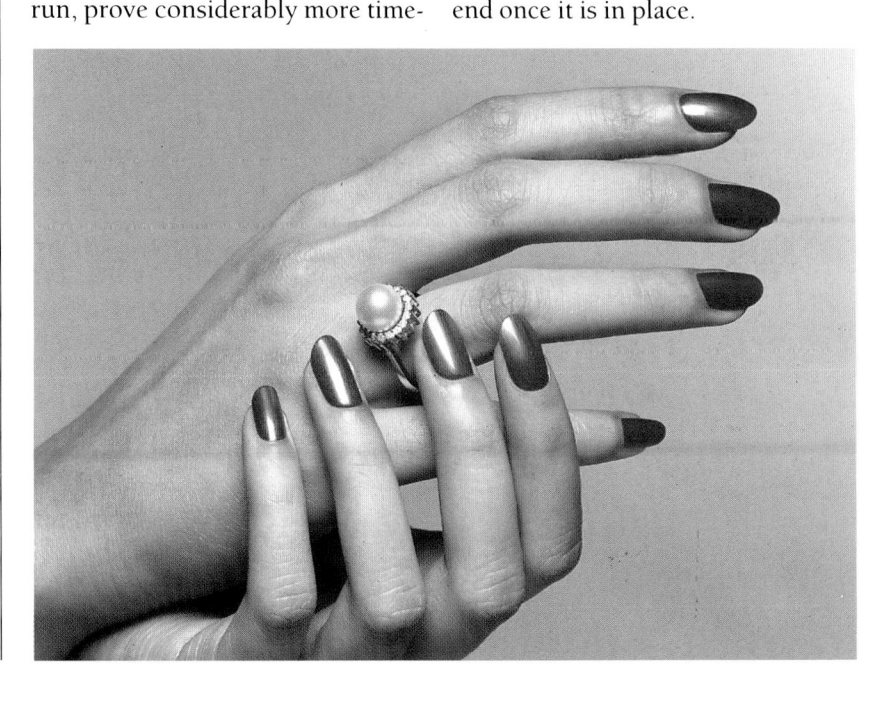

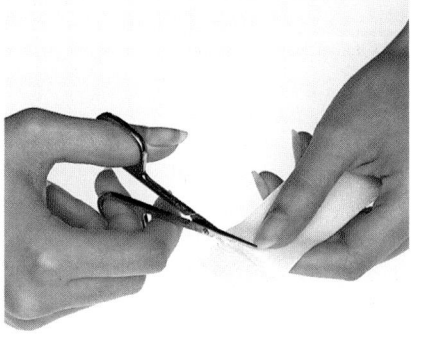

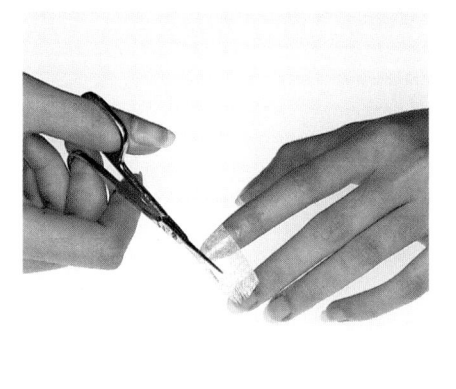

1 *Having buffed your nail with a medium weight buffer, cut a strip of the wrap to the required length with scissors.*

2 *Apply it to your nail and cut to fit the natural shape.*

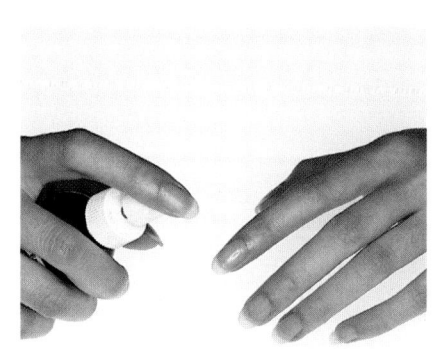

3 *Attach the wrap to the nail with two coats of glue.*

4 *Spray with activator spray, and then buff, work through all the sections on a three-way buffer, until smooth and shiny.*

REPAIRS WITH WRAPS

What you need
Glue
Activator spray
Nail wrap
Nail buffer

If you find yourself with a split nail and a long wait before you can get to your manicure kit, you may need something stronger than glue to fix the damage. Even quite badly broken nails can be salvaged with the aid of a fiberglass wrap. Glue plus a wrap is preferable to glue on its own, and likely to last far longer. However, it is a fiddly procedure which requires a steady hand and total concentration. Wash your hands and remove any nail polish before you begin.

Apply glue to the broken nail and allow it to dry first, then fix the wrap to the nail. The final buffing should be very thorough, to smooth out any tell-tale ridges. This is important, because polish applied on an uneven surface chips very easily. One disadvantage of wrapping is that a close look at the finished nail reveals a fine mesh, which clear polish does not hide. However, the palest of opaque polishes will easily obscure it if you apply two coats.

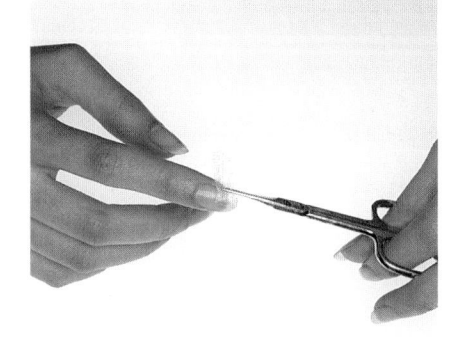

1 *Apply glue to break (see page 28), and buff lightly.*

2 *Once the glue has dried, cut a thin strip of nail wrap and apply to break.*

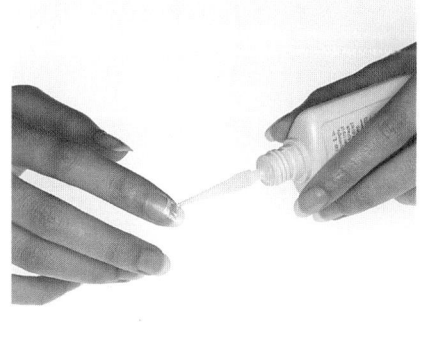

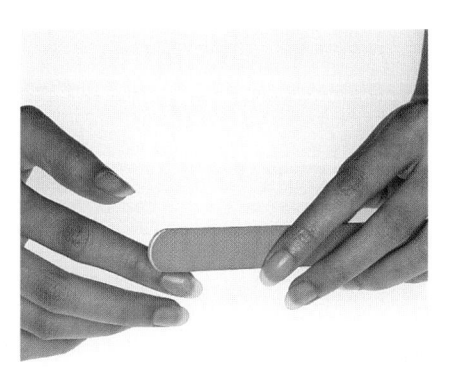

3 *Apply glue, and spray with activator spray, holding it at least 6" (15.5cms) away from your hand.*

4 *Buff nail with three-way buffer, first using the rough side, and then the lighter side, until the nail is smooth and shiny.*

ARTIFICIAL NAILS

What you need
Artificial nail(s)
Glue
Activator spray
Nail buffer
Nail polish

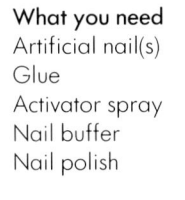

Artificial nails are very useful if you have broken a single nail and don't want to have to file down the other nine to match it, and a lot of fun if you want a set of long scarlet temptress's talons to carry off a party outfit. Also, if you are a compulsive nail biter it may be that the simplest way to remove temptation is to cover your nails over with false ones. Protected, they will have a chance to grow and, perhaps, when the plastic comes off, pride will prevent you from ever chomping on them again.

Like many cosmetic innovations, artificial nails came from Hollywood, where, in the 1930s, crude plastic replica nails adorned the stars' fingers. Now, they are far more sophisticated, and, if applied carefully and polished, can look just like the real thing.

False nails "grow" with the real nail, leaving a gap at the base after about two weeks, which will need filling. This can be tricky and is usually best left to a manicurist.

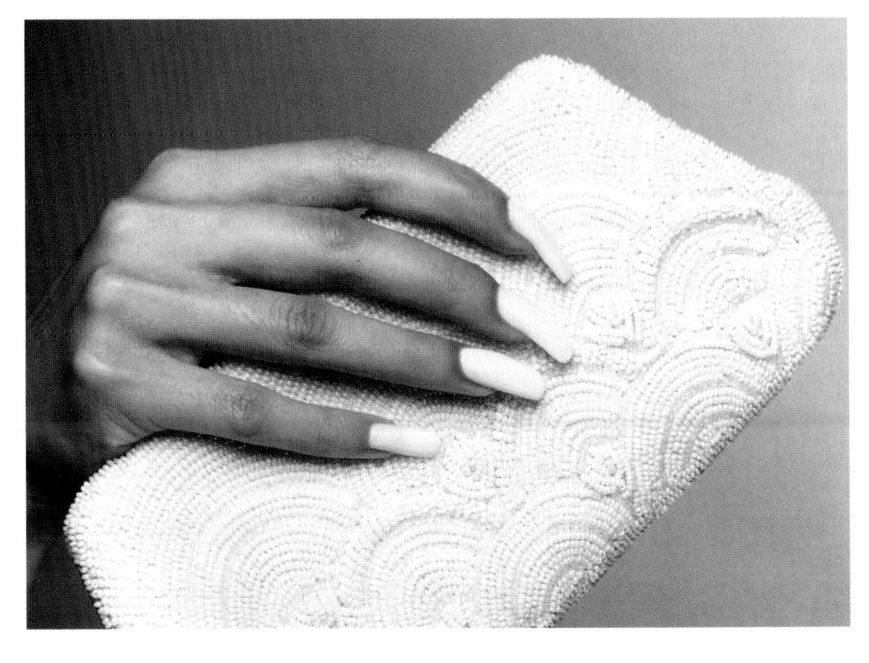

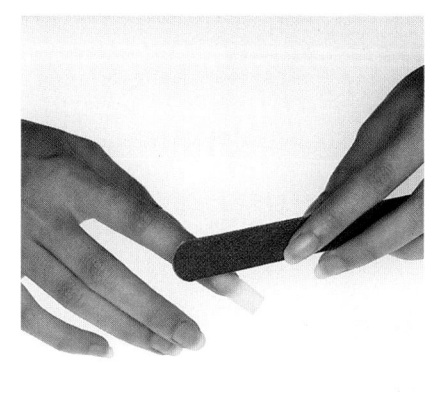

1 *After buffing your nail, select a suitably sized artificial nail, apply glue to the underside, and attach to natural nail.*

2 *Blend the artificial nail into your own with a light weight file until the join disappears. File into the desired shape.*

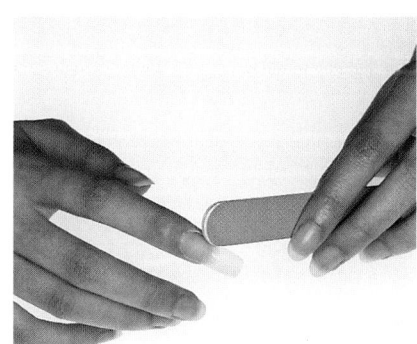

3 *Apply glue over the entire surface and spray with activator spray.*

4 *Buff with a three-way buffer and apply polish.*

DECORATED NAILS

What you need
Artificial nail(s)
Nail polish
Glue
Activator spray
Nail buffer
Top coat
Strip of thin, flexible
   material such as
   aluminum foil

With a set of false nails and a steady hand, the possibilities for decoration are endless – black and white motifs, stars and stripes, Christmas trees, and practically any other festive or personalized variation can be achieved with some perseverence.

Good quality polish is vital; it must be easy to apply, have an even consistency and color, and be very long lasting. Whether or not you intend to decorate your nails with patterns, it is worth shopping around for reliable polish – as with many other cosmetic products, price is usually a good indication of quality.

If you find painting your nails difficult, these effects will take some practice. Try it on one hand only at first.

Painting a stripe straight onto a nail is very difficult, and it is far easier to paint something else and then apply it to the nail afterwards. Here, we have used a metallic strip, and finished with a clear top coat.

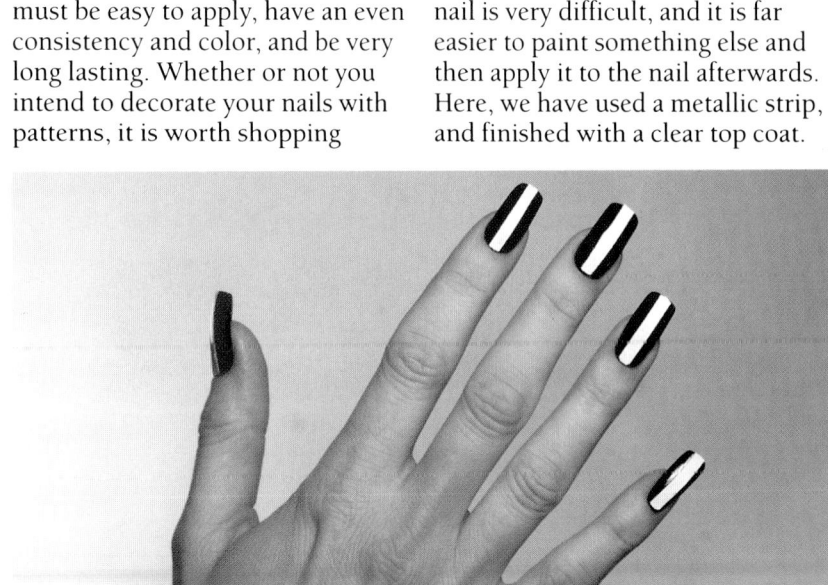

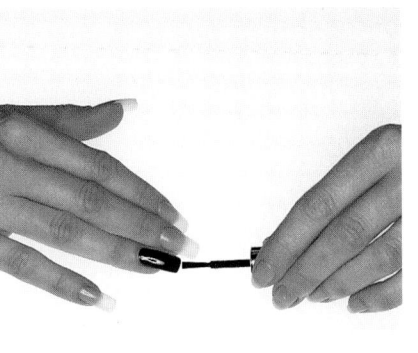

1 *Apply false nail (see page 42), filing it into the desired shape.*

2 *Apply black nail polish with brush (see page 32).*

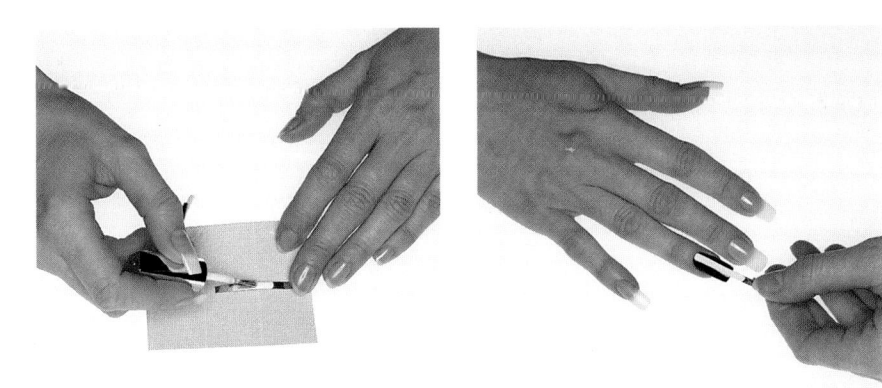

3 *Paint metallic strip with white polish. Single strokes will give the best finish. Leave until completely dry.*

4 *Attach white strip to nail with glue before applying a clear top coat.*

SUMMER HANDS

What you need
Almond oil
Nail polish remover
Moisturizer
Base coat
Nail polish

As soon as the weather hots up, we apply sunscreen religiously to our faces and bodies – but the backs of our hands, the most exposed areas of all, tend to go unprotected. It is true that hands rarely get sunburnt in the way that shoulders and legs do, but the back of the hand is one of the places where skin cancer may develop, particularly if you live in a very hot climate.

Hands also age faster than any other part of the body, and there is little you can do about it. As well as causing premature ageing, too much sun can make liver spots appear on the backs of hands. These can be minimized by applying lemon juice (see page 9).

It is also thought that the sun may weaken and damage the nails themselves, so if you are not wearing polish to go to the beach, it is a good idea to put some sunscreen on them at the same time as you do your hands. Soaking your fingertips in almond oil will help to keep the cuticles soft and the nails flexible.

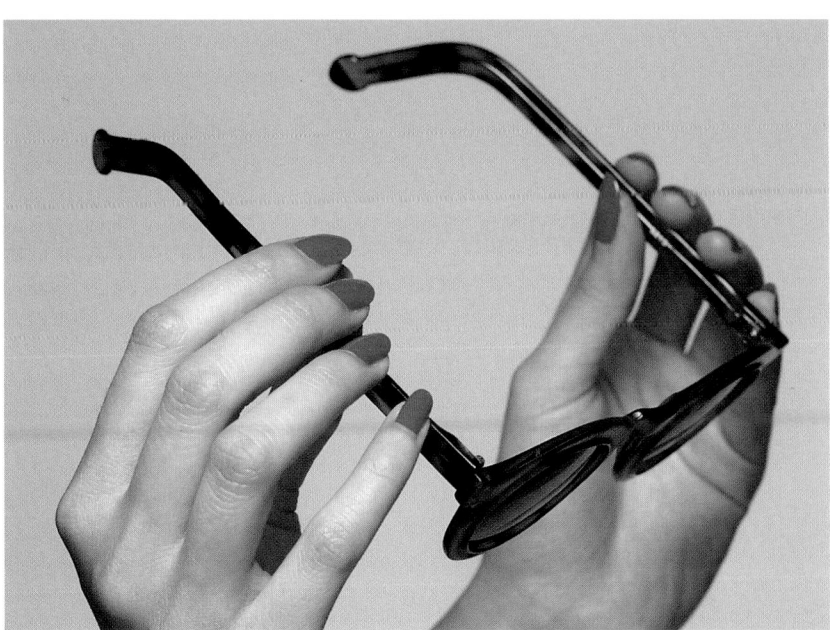

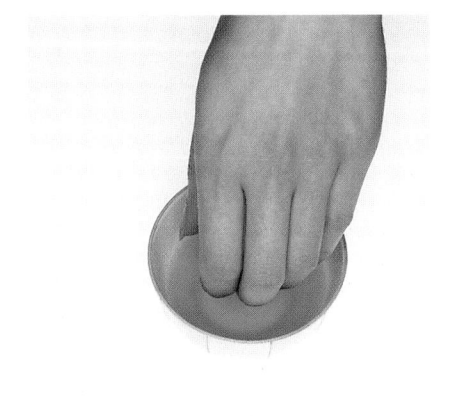

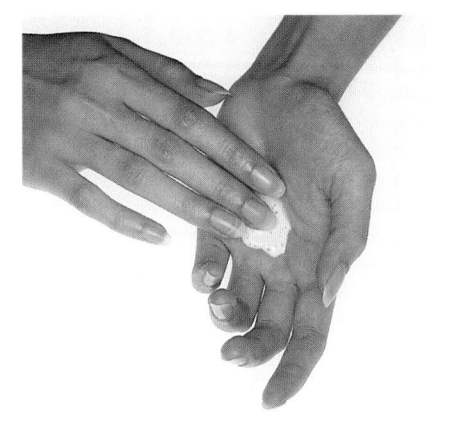

1 *Soak your nails in almond oil, and before painting remove all excess oil.*

2 *Massage hands thoroughly using a moisturizer, preferably with added sunscreen. Make sure that it is rubbed in well.*

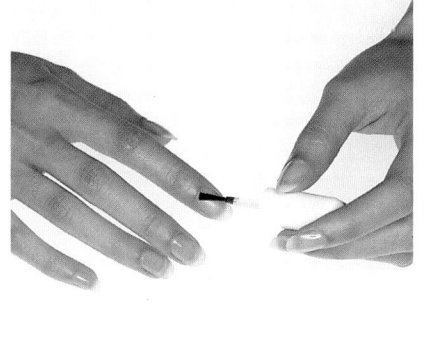

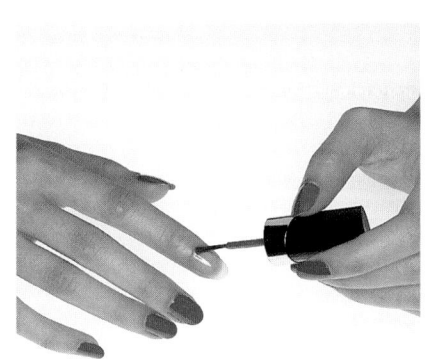

3 *Apply base coat to protect your nails and help prevent polish chipping.*

4 *Apply colored polish to suit your mood or the occasion.*

WINTER HANDS

What you need
Exfoliant
Hand mask (or face
    mask)
Moisturizer

In winter, hands can get very dry, rough and sore. Washing them will make them rougher still, so do it gently, and try to avoid scrubbing at your nails with a hard brush. Aggressive scrubbing will certainly weaken your nails, and it may force the nail plate up and away from the nail bed (see diagram on page 7).

To protect your hands from chapping, take extra care to dry them thoroughly after washing. It will also help the skin to stay supple and well-nourished if you keep a heavy-duty moisturizer by the sink for an application after every wash.

Try to avoid exposing your hands to harsh, biting winds, because this can leave them very sore indeed. Invest in several pairs of winter gloves that match your clothes.

Poor circulation can lead to unattractive, mottled, pink and purple fingers, and blue nails. A vigorous massage will help improve the flow of blood to the hands generally and to the nail bed (see page 64), restoring a healthy glow.

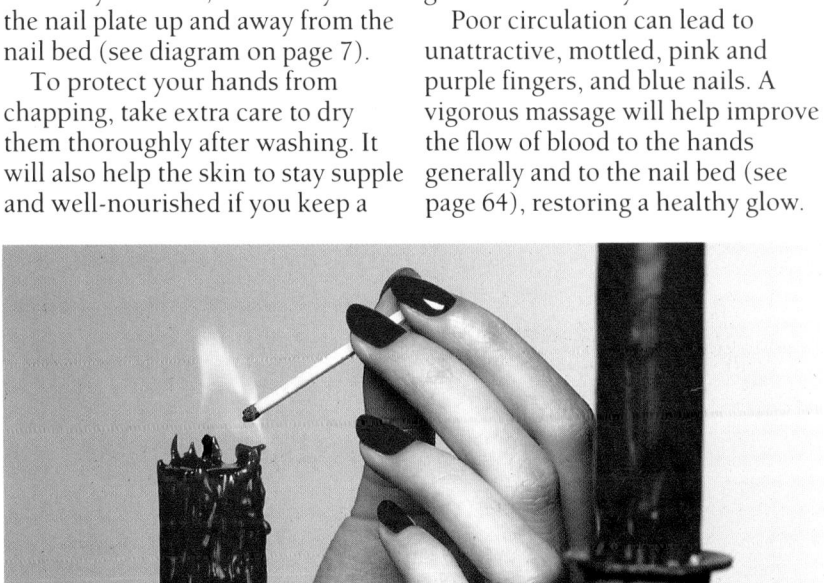

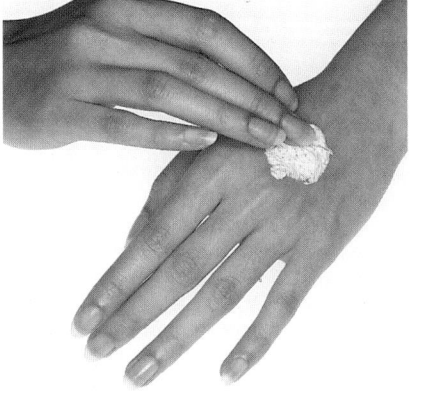

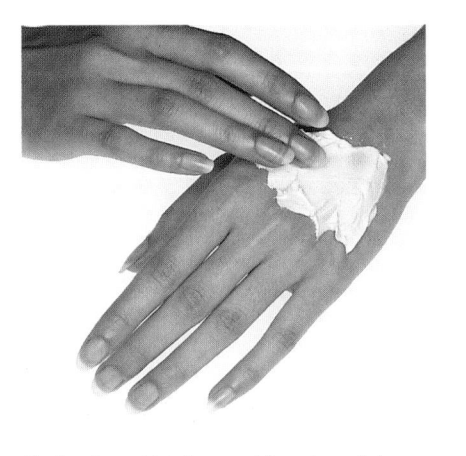

1 *Apply a small amount of exfoliant with circular motions of your finger. Then wash your hands and dry thoroughly.*

2 *Apply a thick layer of hand mask (see page 15).*

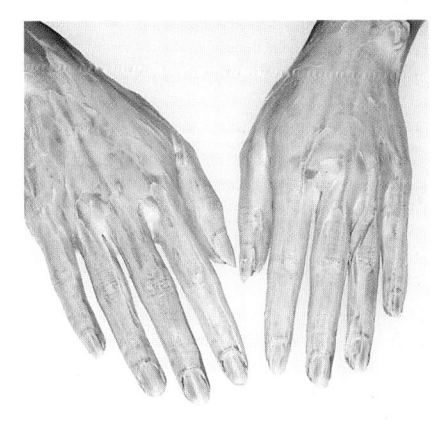

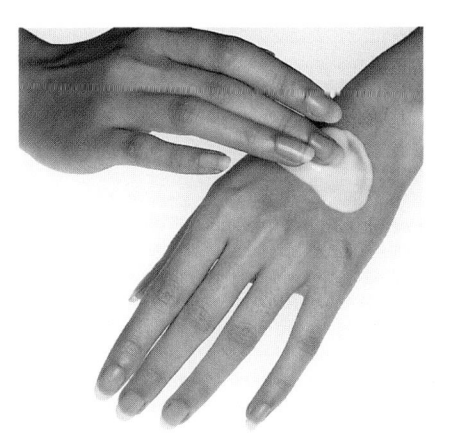

3 *Keep the hand mask on for as long as possible.*

4 *Apply a rich moisturizer. Work into the skin with a circular motion, as before.*

QUICK MANICURE

What you need
Cotton ball
Nail polish remover
Shallow bowl
Orange stick
Base coat

If your nail polish needs changing, or you've had a hard day and want to pamper yourself, why not give your hands a treat by incorporating this simple manicure into your beauty routine?

Try to choose a non-acetone polish remover, and apply it with a cotton ball or pad. Hold the cotton ball down on your nail for a few seconds to dissolve the polish, then rub it off with a stroking movement from the base of your nail to the tip. Use a fresh cotton ball for each nail.

If you don't own a special manicurist's bath, it doesn't matter: a soup bowl will do just as well. Fill it with warm soapy water.

Wrap some cotton around the end of your orange stick before attending to your cuticles – never poke at them with anything sharp.

One layer of base coat should be enough to protect your nails, provided you aren't planning to go coal mining or mountaineering! For the evening, you can apply colored polish straight over it.

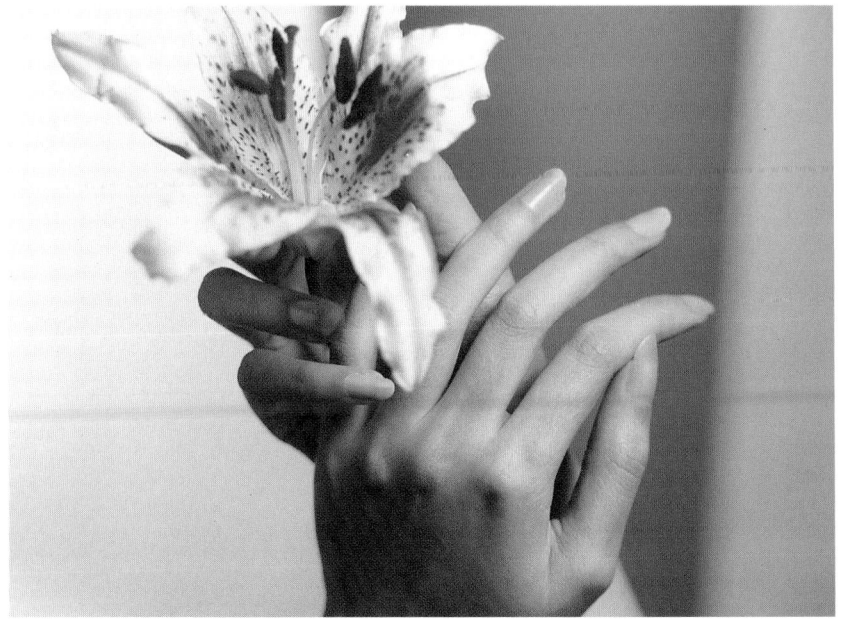

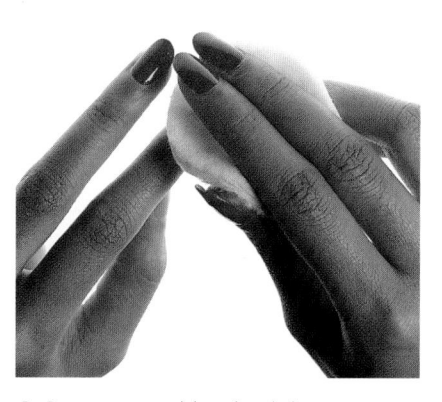

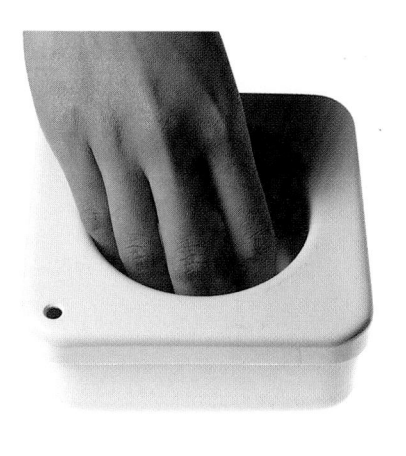

1 *Remove any old nail polish using a cotton ball or pad.*

2 *Soak your nails. Allow at least one minute for each hand.*

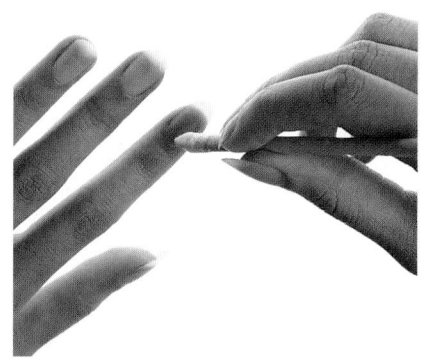

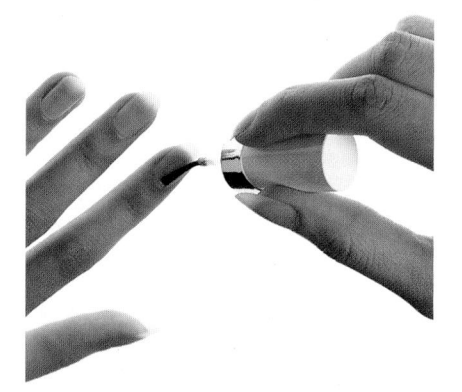

3 *Push back your cuticles gently with an orange stick. Do not force them.*

4 *Paint your nails with a base coat before applying a colored polish.*

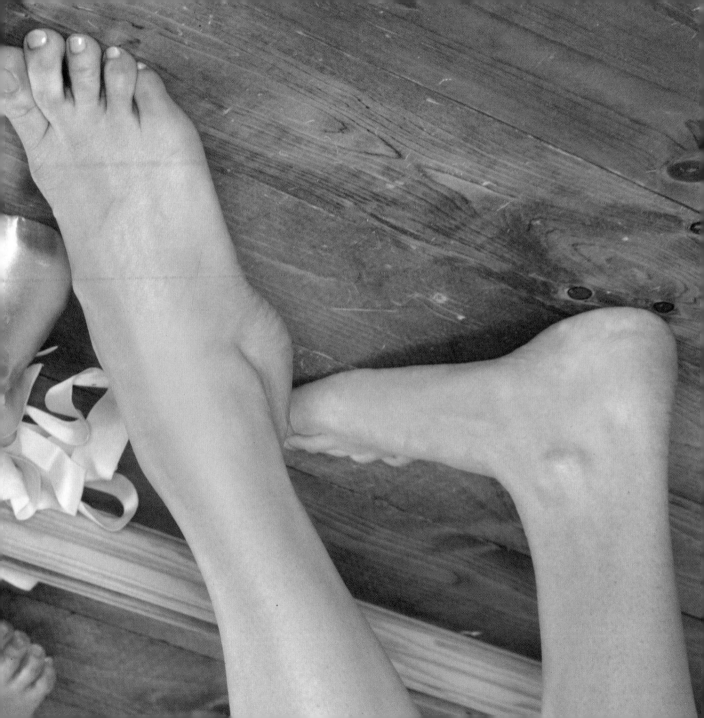

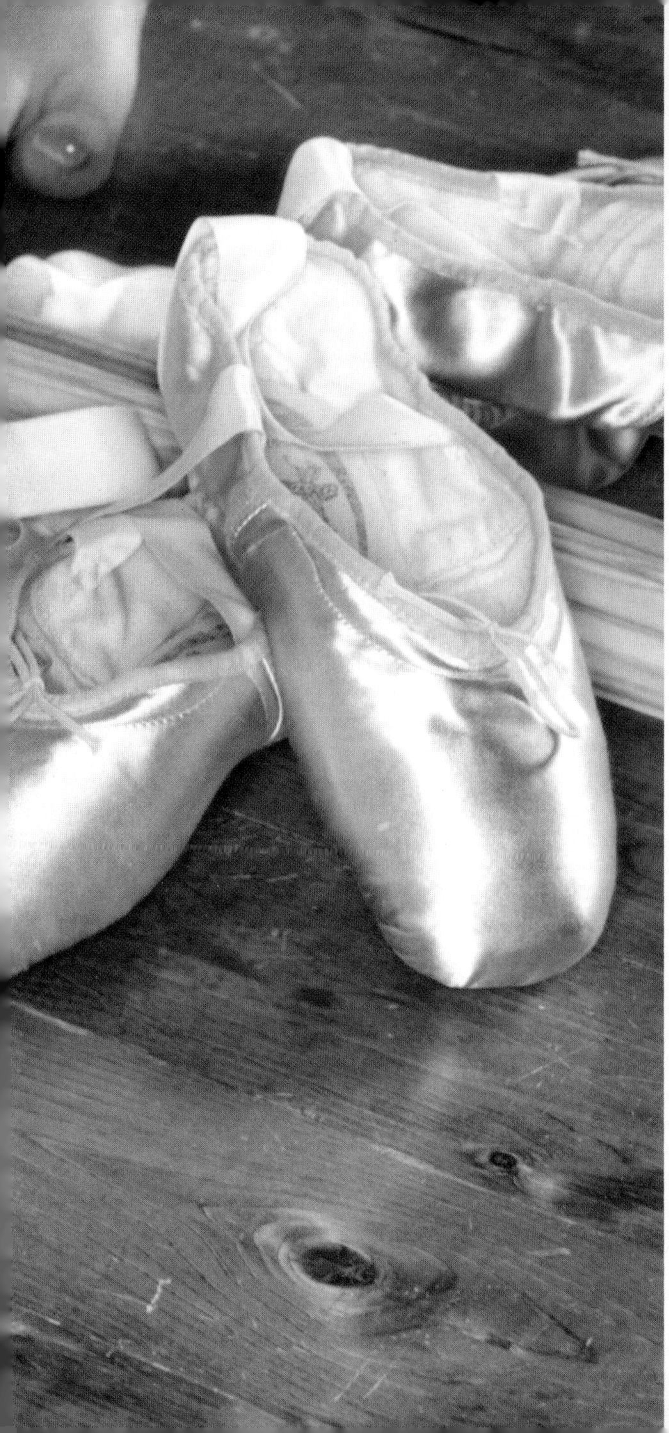

2
PEDICURES

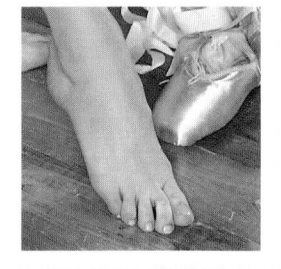

Skin softener

What you need
Bowl of warm soapy
water
Metal file or pumice
stone
Medium weight
(plastic) file
Body lotion

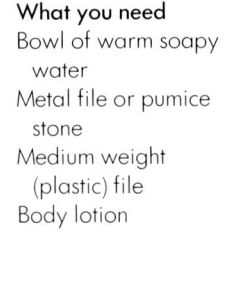

Feet take a lot of punishment from high heels, tight shoes, synthetic fabrics and sidewalk pounding, so it is hardly surprising that they develop areas of rough skin and calluses. Hard skin needs to be tackled regularly with a special file or pumice stone in order to keep it down. If you have a big build-up of hard skin, you should see a chiropodist rather than trying to remove it yourself.

If your feet are aching, try giving them a soothing soak in warm water with added bath salts. When you are drying your feet, take the opportunity to inspect them for any problems such as corns or athlete's foot. Be especially careful about drying thoroughly between your toes, as bacteria can breed far more easily in this area if it is moist.

When you rub in a skin softening cream, massage all the areas of your feet as thoroughly as possible: your sole, heel, and instep, as well as the top of your foot and your ankle (see page 70).

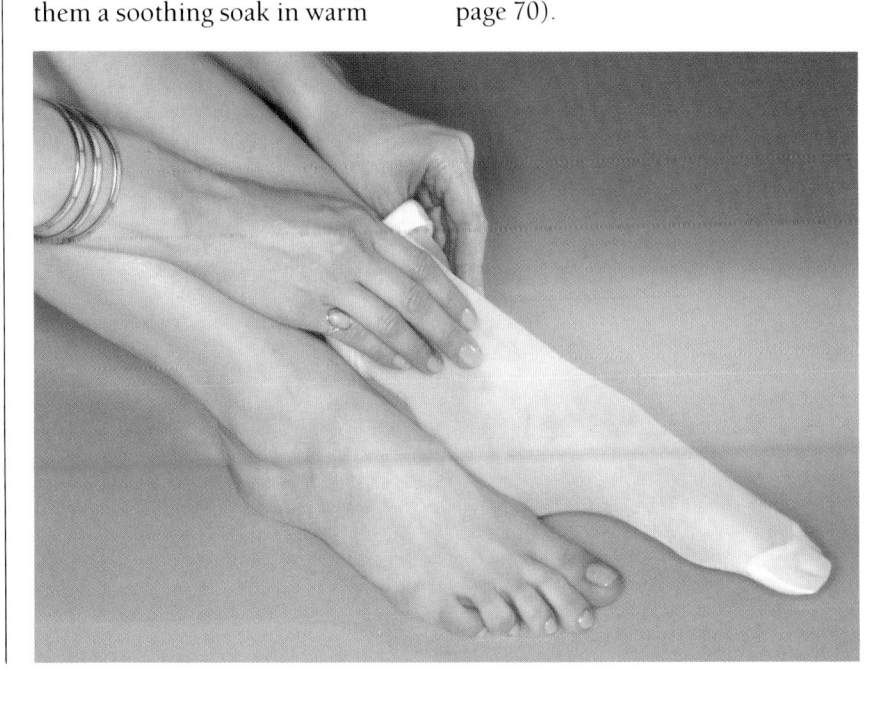

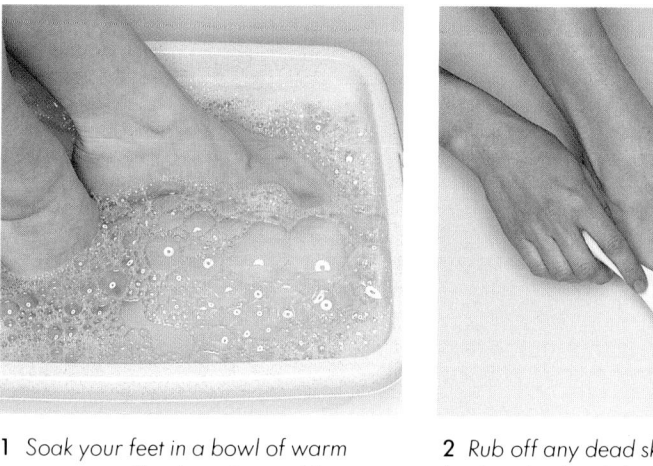

1 Soak your feet in a bowl of warm soapy water. Dry them thoroughly.

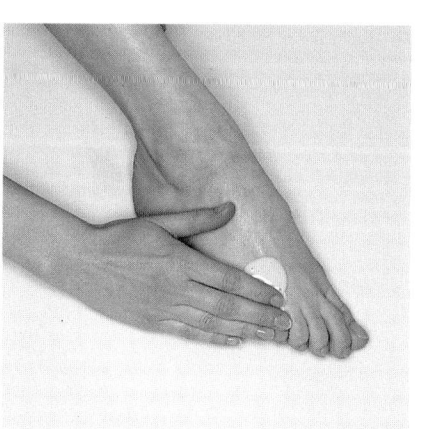

2 Rub off any dead skin around your heels with a hard skin remover like this metal one, or a pumice stone.

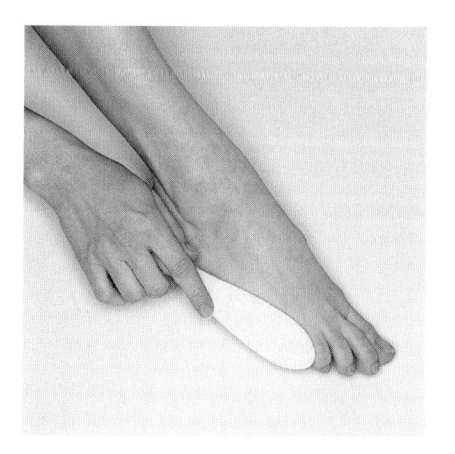

3 Smooth the area off with a medium weight file, like the plastic one here.

4 Rub hand cream or body lotion into your feet, especially around the heels.

Trimming toenails

What you need
Toenail clippers
Nail file

Although toenails tend to grow considerably more slowly than fingernails, they are not subjected to the same kinds of wear and tear, so they do need to be trimmed regularly. Over-long toenails, as well as being a menace to tights and stockings, can make shoes very uncomfortable; and constant jabbing against the inside of a shoe can, in time, lead to a bruised and sore toenail.

Be careful not to cut or file your nails right back into the corners, as this can cause ingrowing toenails (see page 18). As they can become quite hard and horny, toenails should be cut with clippers designed for the purpose, not with nail scissors or fingernail clippers. A pair of scissors that isn't up to the job will tear and splinter the nails, so it is worth investing in some decent clippers.

A medium weight nail file is shown here, but if your toenails are really tough, you may need to use something stronger.

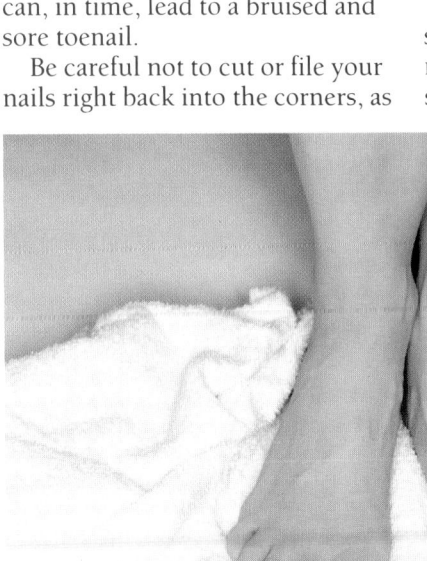

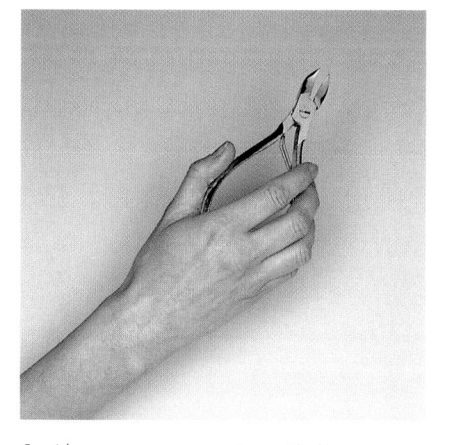

1 *Always use proper toenail clippers, like the ones shown.*

2 *Cut toenails straight across with clippers in a single motion, taking care not to make them too short.*

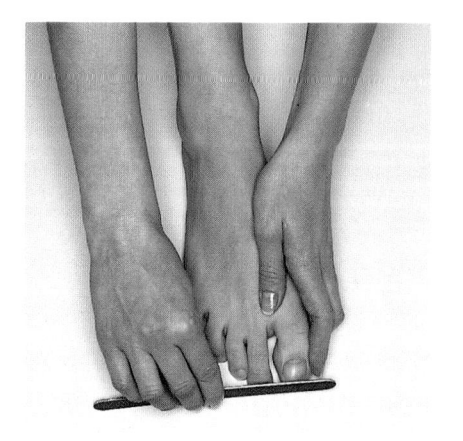

3 *File nails straight across with a medium-weight file.*

QUICK PEDICURE

What you need
Nail file
Toenail clippers
Cuticle cream
Hoof stick or orange
    stick
Exfoliant
Body lotion

Feet tend to be neglected in favor of hands, simply because we don't see our unshod feet as often. Over winter, encased in thick tights and stout shoes for most of the time, our feet often receive no attention at all. However, tired, sore feet should never be ignored, because they can be the harbinger of a whole series of health problems.

If you want to give your feet a much deserved pick-me-up, this pedicure is an ideal way to do it. The best time is after a bath, when your feet will have had a good soak. The cuticles on your toenails serve the same purpose as those on your hands, and should be treated with equal respect. Use a rubber tipped hoof stick or an orange stick wrapped in cotton to push cuticles back. You can also push gently with the towel, when drying your feet. When you rub in the hand cream, avoid the areas directly between your toes; these should be kept as dry as possible so as not to encourage fungal infections.

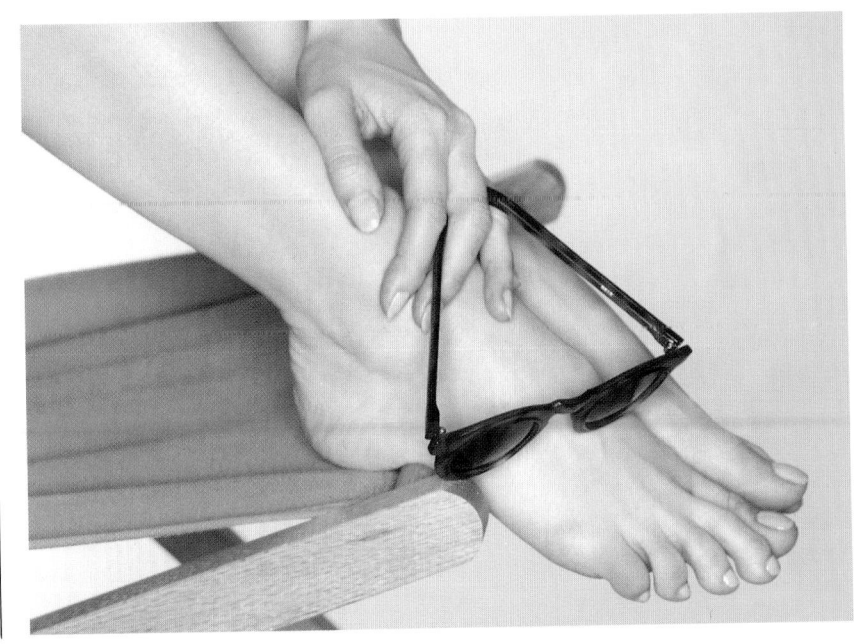

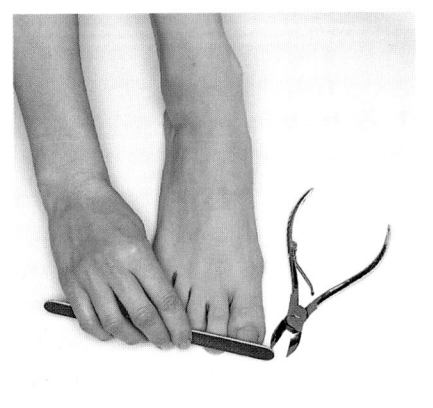

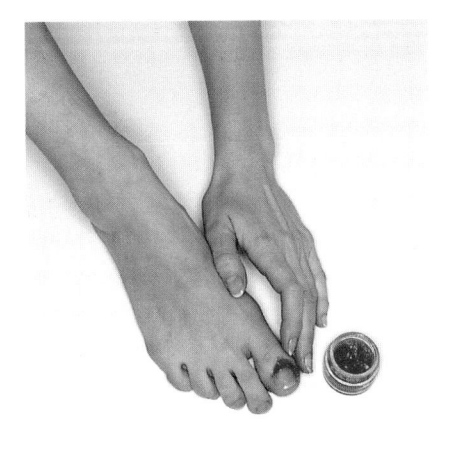

1 Clip your toenails straight across, and file smooth with an emery board (see page 56).

2 Apply cuticle cream and rub well in with the balls of your thumbs.

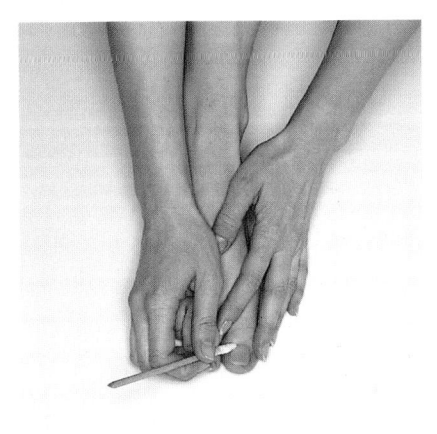

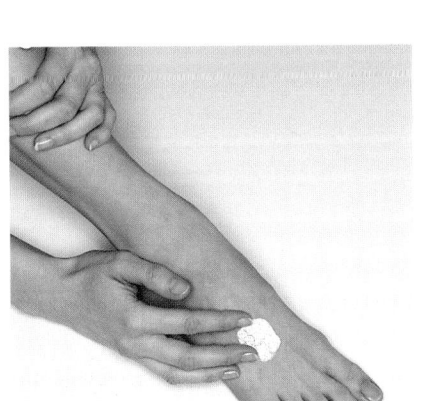

3 Push back your cuticles with a hoof stick or cotton wrapped orange stick.

4 Apply exfoliant with circular motions of your fingers. Rinse your feet and dry thoroughly. Rub in body lotion.

PAINTING TOENAILS

What you need
Separator or cotton balls
Base coat
Nail polish
Top coat

Painted toenails take a notoriously long time to dry. For a really professional effect, paint your nails when you know you won't need to wear shoes for a couple of hours. If you only leave them for ten minutes before stuffing them into shoes, the polish will smudge.

Your toenail polish needs to match your shoes, outfit, and finger nails – scarlet toenails, however beautifully painted, will look unbalanced if they are matched with frosted pink fingernails (although natural or pale toenails will coordinate with any color fingernail). If you have slender, straight toes, then a bright color will enhance them. However, if they are not your best feature, try a clear or pale colored polish.

Before you start, make sure that any old polish has been thoroughly removed. If it is difficult to remove the varnish around the cuticle with an ordinary cotton ball, tease out a portion of the cotton ball and wrap it around an orange stick.

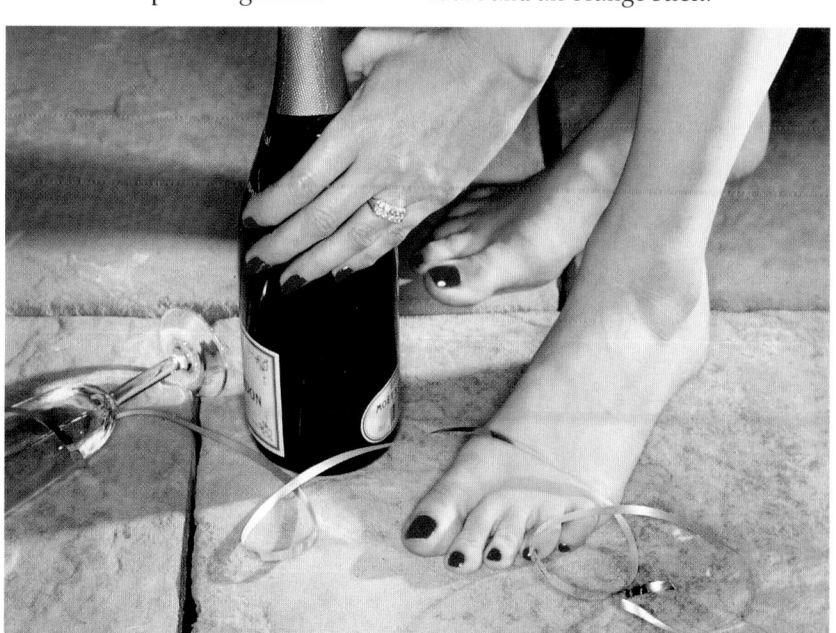

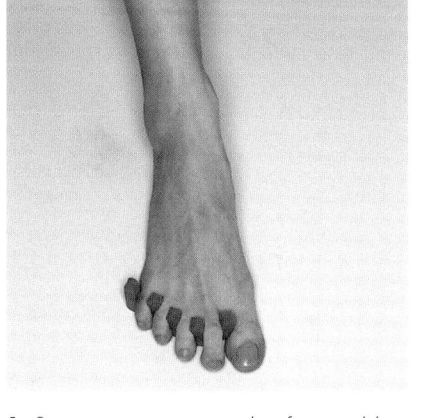

1 *Separate your toes with a foam rubber separator. If you do not have one, cotton balls will do.*

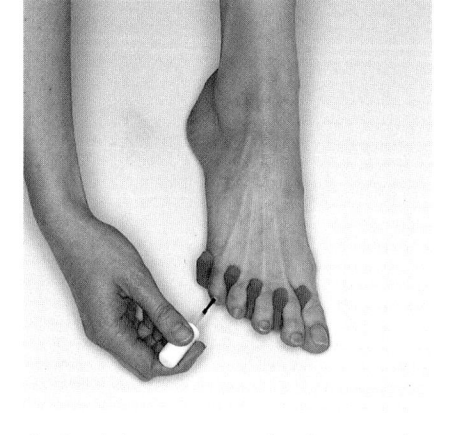

2 *Apply base coat as a first layer, and leave to dry.*

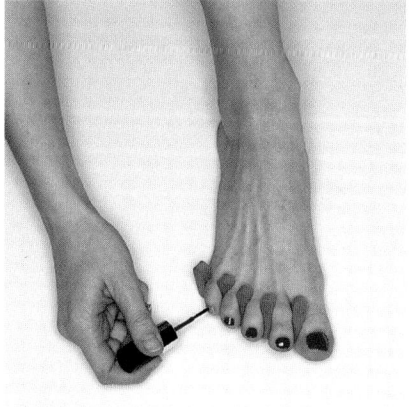

3 *Apply two coats of colored polish and leave to dry.*

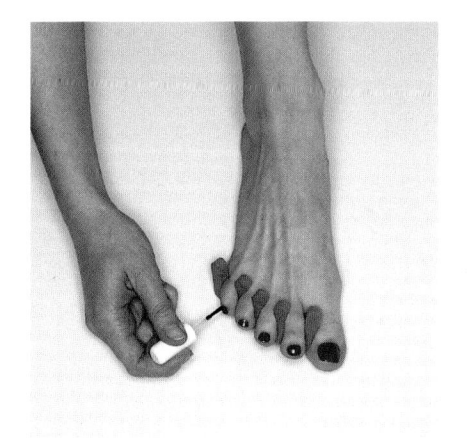

4 *Apply top coat. Leave to dry thoroughly before putting on shoes.*

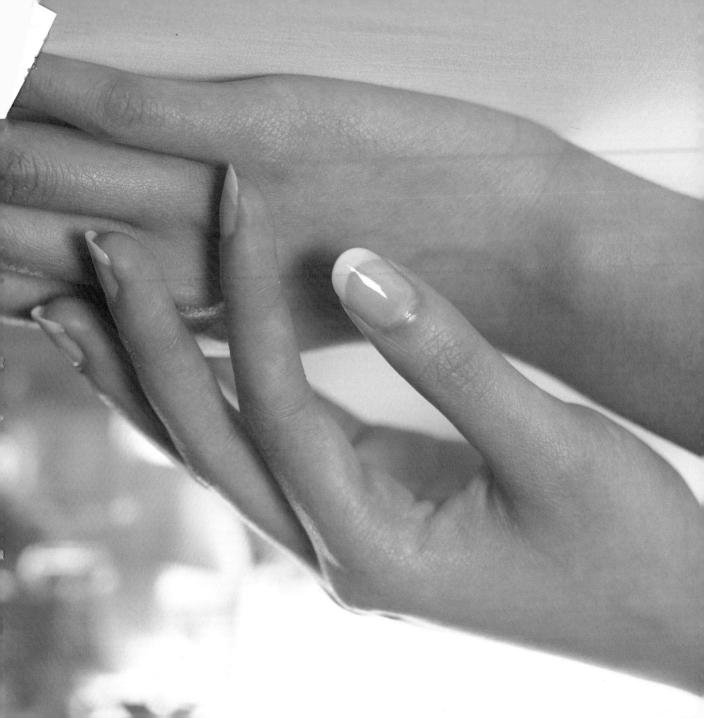

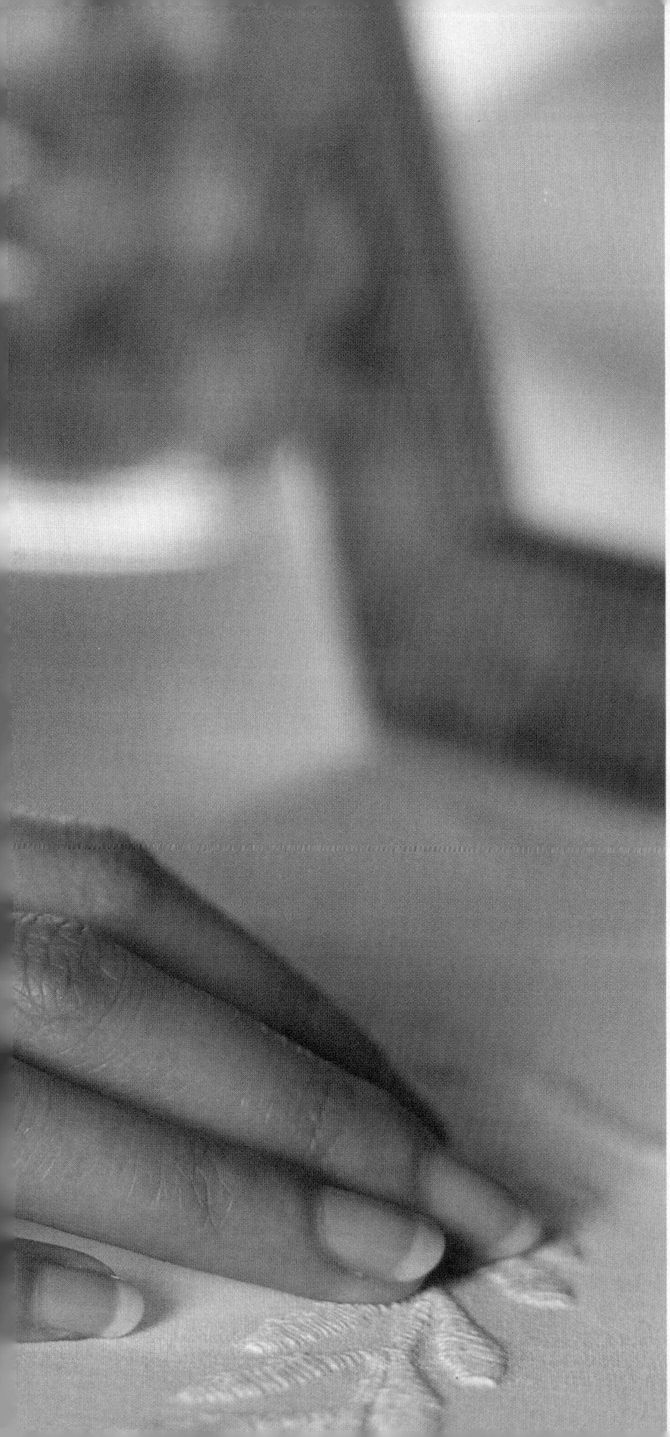

3
MASSAGES AND
EXERCISES

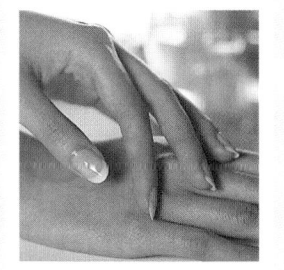

FINGER MASSAGE

What you need
Massage oil

Massage can help to soothe away aches and pains, relieve tension and make you feel relaxed. Of course, it is nicer when there is someone else to massage you, but hands and fingers, unlike shoulders and backs, can be reached more easily by their owners.

Establish a smooth rhythm, and go lightly over any areas where the bones are near the surface of the skin, such as the backs of the hands. The metacarpals, which are the bones of your hand, are quite near the surface, so take care not to dig into them too hard with your thumb.

There are plenty of rich massage oils available, but if you don't have any, olive oil from the kitchen will do. Apply it liberally – you can always wipe off the excess afterwards with a paper towel.

Don't give yourself a hand or finger massage if you suffer from arthritis, rheumatism or swollen and painful fingers, as you will probably do more harm than good.

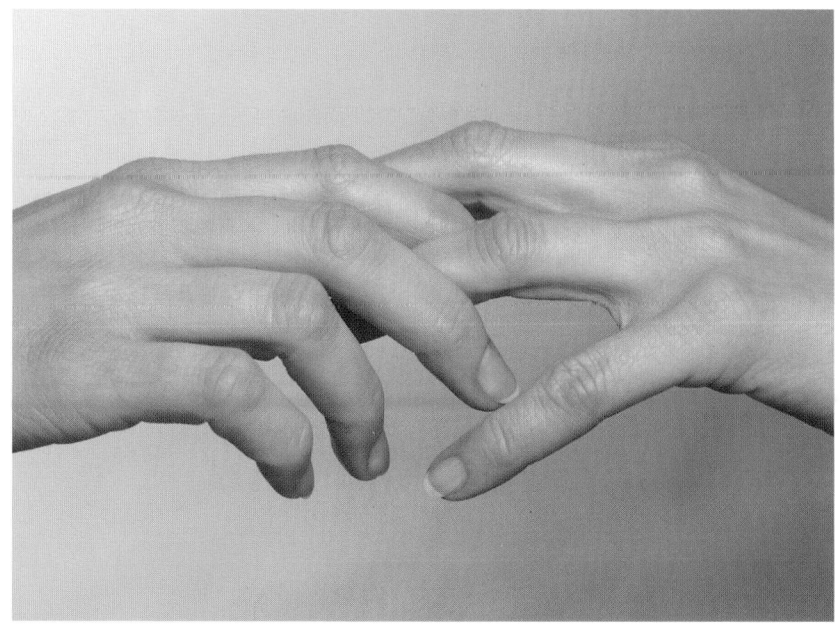

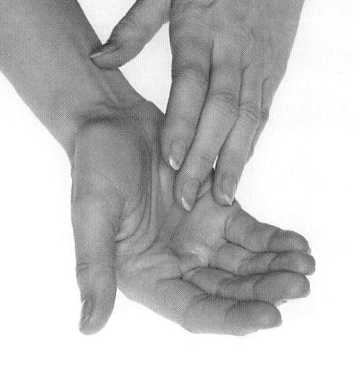

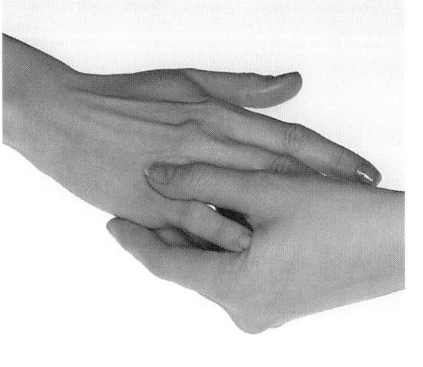

1 *Pour a small amount of massage oil into your palm.*

2 *Massage between metacarpals with the thumb of your other hand, using a circular motion.*

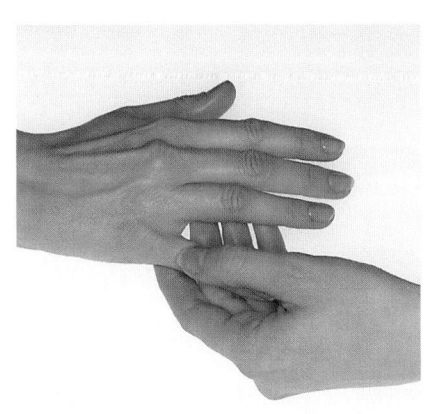

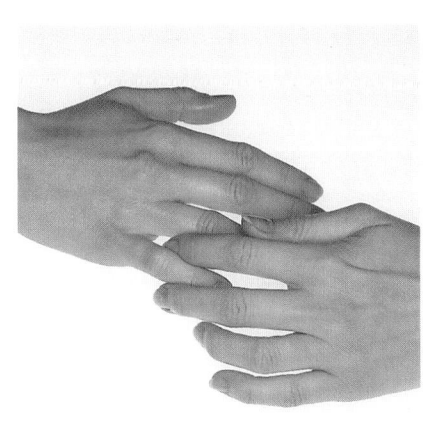

3 *Massage, using the same circular motion of the thumb, down the length of each finger.*

4 *'Scissor' your fingers with the first and second fingers of the other hand, using a firm backwards pulling motion.*

PALM AND ARM MASSAGE

What you need
Massage oil

Regular massaging helps to improve your skin tone and texture by increasing the circulation of the blood directly beneath the skin. When applying pressure on the hand and arm, as in steps 3 and 4 shown here, always move upwards, towards your heart.

There are three different massage strokes. *Effleurage* is a soothing, stroking movement with the fingertips, or, on larger areas, the palm of the hand. *Pettrissage* is a deeper movement for relieving tension. As when kneading bread dough, the tissues are pressed and then relaxed. *Friction* is a circular movement of the thumbs which stimulates the circulation and releases 'knotted' muscles.

If you are concerned about the state of the skin on your hands, try to put in a few minutes of massage every time after drying them, especially in the winter. You will be helping to prevent dryness and chilblains as well as improving your skin tone.

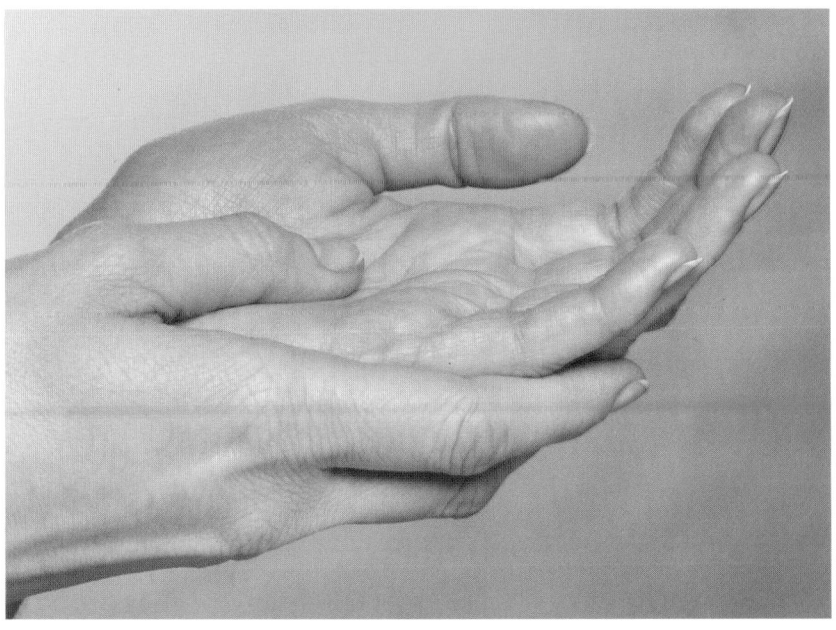

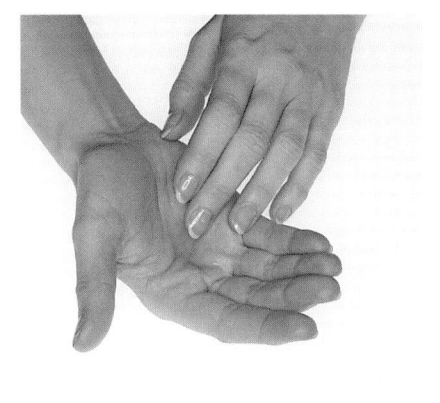

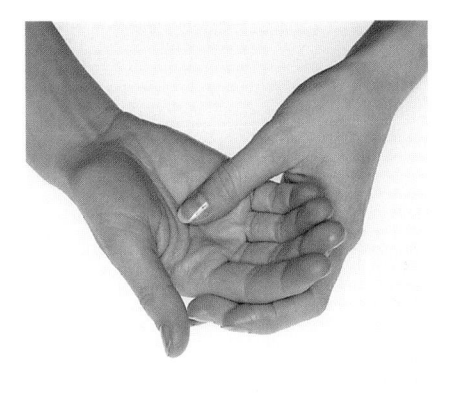

1 *Pour a small amount of massage oil into your palm.*

2 *Massage your palm with the thumb of your other hand in a circular motion.*

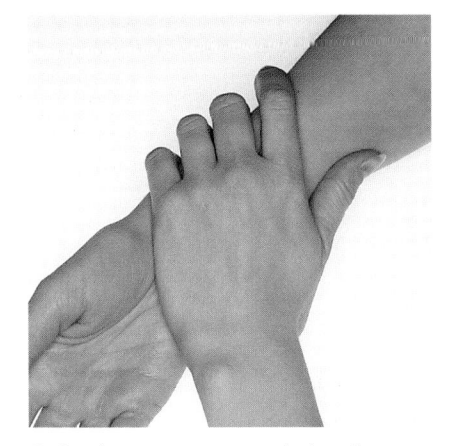

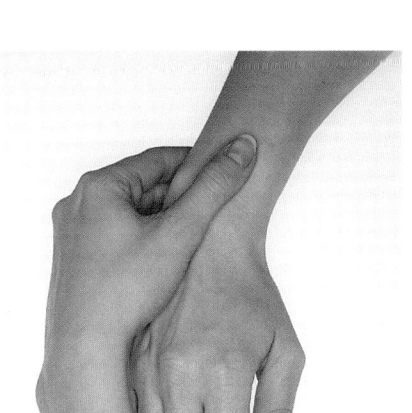

3 *Stroke your arm towards the elbow, using firm upward movements, lifting your hand away each time.*

4 *Rub your forearm from wrist to elbow with firm circular movements of the thumb.*

EXERCISES FOR HANDS

What you need
Comfortable chair

If you find yourself with a spare moment, a few simple hand exercises will improve flexibility and circulation. Manipulating joints loosens them up and increases their suppleness.

Hand exercises do not require any special equipment, and they don't work up a sweat, so you can do them anywhere. Here are a couple to add to your exercise routine: rest the tips of your fingers lightly on a firm surface, such as a table, and drum with your fingers, quite quickly, as if you are impatient. Then, removing your hands from the table, clench both your fists tightly, and then open up your hands, stretching out your fingers to their fullest extent. Repeat this ten times.

A good way to start and finish your hand exercises is to stand with your arms hanging loosely by your sides, allowing your hands and wrists to relax and go completely limp. Then give them a good shake until they are tingling.

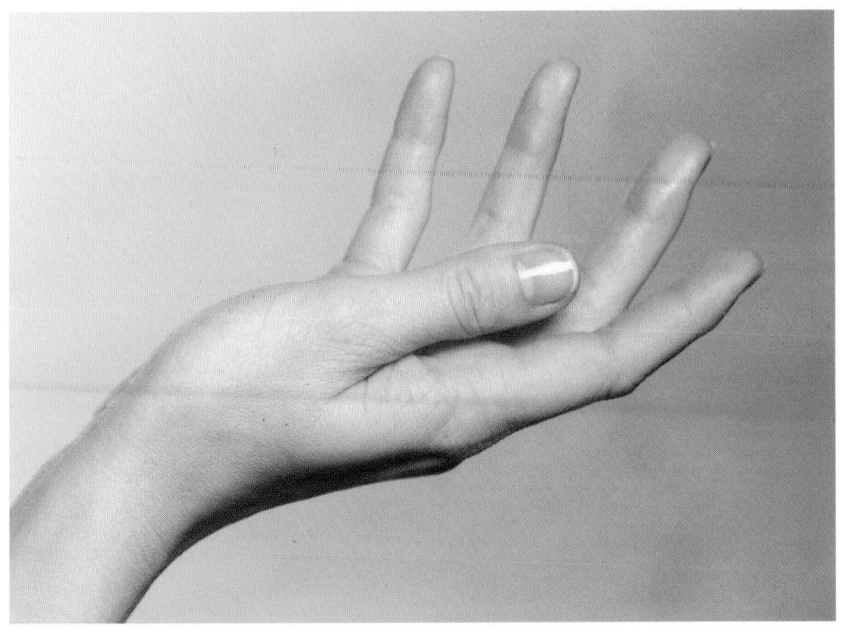

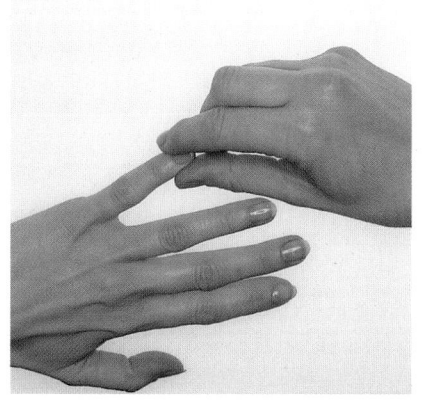

1 *Rotate each finger three times in each direction, manipulating it between the thumb and first finger of your other hand.*

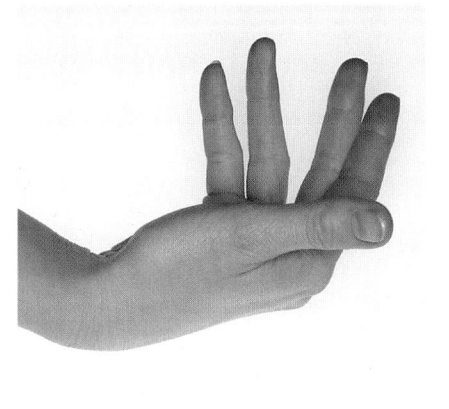

2 *Rotate your wrists gently, first in one direction and then the other.*

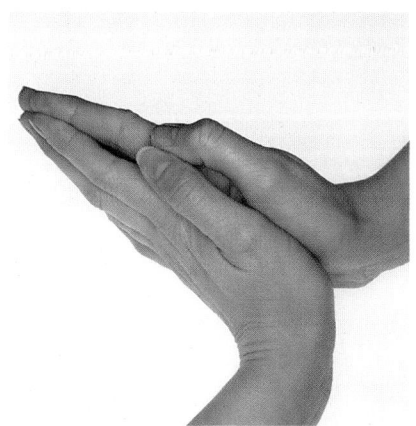

3 *Bend wrist backwards by pressing the heel of your other hand against the palm.*

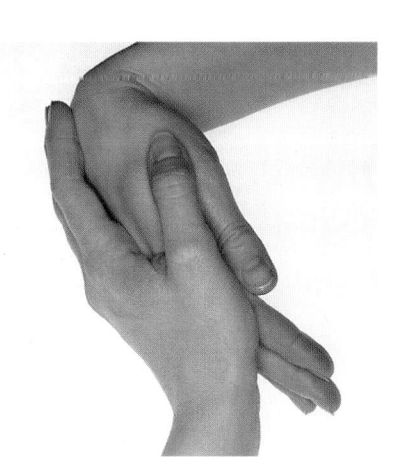

4 *Bend wrist downwards by pressing the palm of your other hand against the back of the hand.*

FOOT AND LOWER LEG MASSAGE

What you need
Massage oil

A massage can work wonders on tired, aching feet, and it is an excellent way to relieve stress. Here's one that you can do yourself. Give your feet a quick wash, dry them thoroughly, and make sure you are sitting in a comfortable position – there's no sense in massaging your feet and straining your back at the same time.

Although a massage can give you a great feeling of well-being, it is not a substitute for exercise, and it cannot reduce fatty deposits in the body. While you are massaging, take a look at your ankles. If they are puffy, it may be due to water retention or bad circulation. There are several things you can do to help this – don't sit with your legs crossed or tucked in underneath your body, as this will cut off the circulation. If you have spent much of the day standing up or pounding the sidewalk, put your feet and ankles in a bowl of hot water for three minutes, followed immediately by cold water.

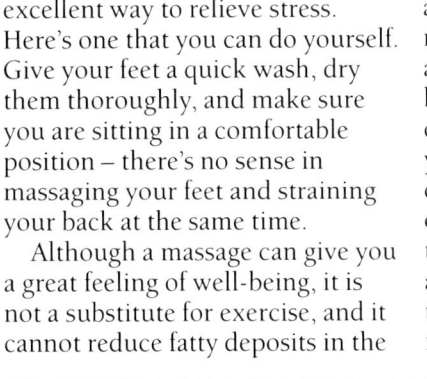

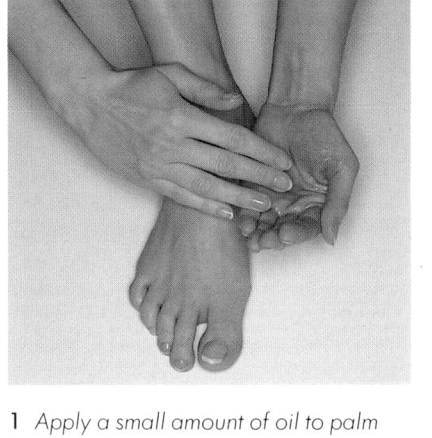

1 *Apply a small amount of oil to palm and spread over both hands.*

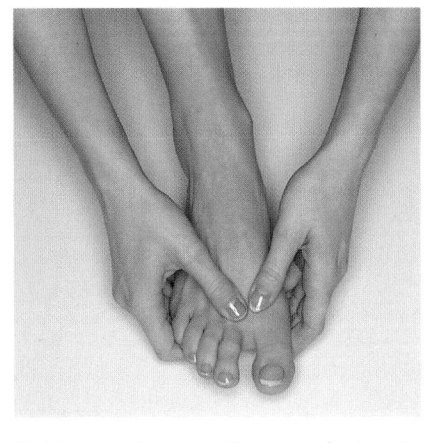

2 *Massage between the metatarsals with both thumbs, using a circular motion.*

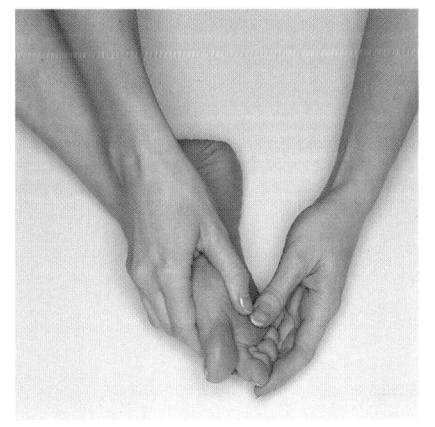

3 *Massage the soles of the feet with both hands, using circular movements.*

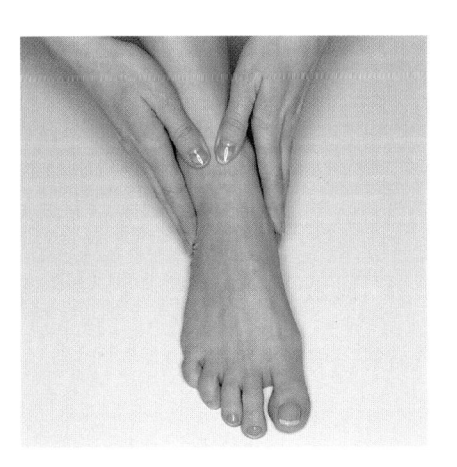

4 *Starting from your ankle, make circular movements with your thumbs, going up towards your knees.*

ANKLE EXERCISES

What you need
Cushion

Ankles vary considerably, and, although exercise cannot turn a thick ankle into a thin one, it is possible to trim off at least some of the fat. Besides looking great, a pair of strong, firm ankles will help to keep your feet in good condition.

Rotating the ankle can be done whenever you're sitting or standing for long periods of time. Anything that relieves the pressure on your ankles is helpful, which is why it is a good idea to finish your exercises by lying down with your feet a little higher than your head. Another exercise which may be helpful is to stand on tiptoe on the edge of a thick book placed on the floor. Keeping your toes in position on the book, and holding onto a chair to prevent you from toppling over, lower your heels to the floor and bring them up again slowly.

Remember that high heels do not necessarily flatter your ankles – heels, especially with an ankle-strap, can have a disastrous effect on thick ankles and calves.

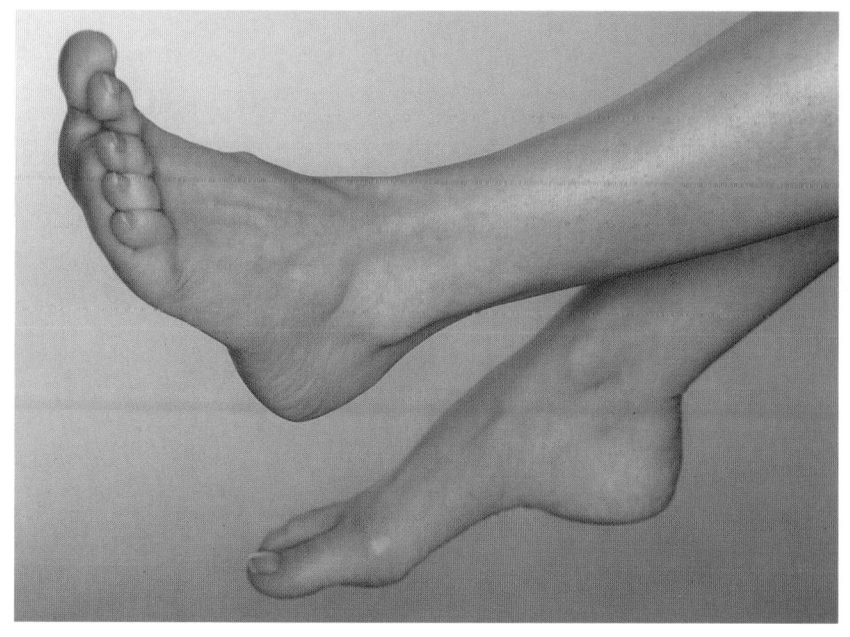

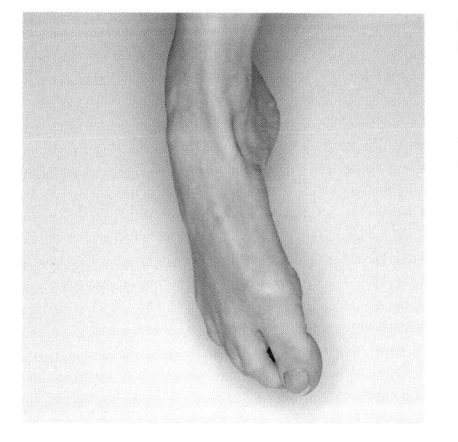

1 Rotate each ankle ten times in each direction.

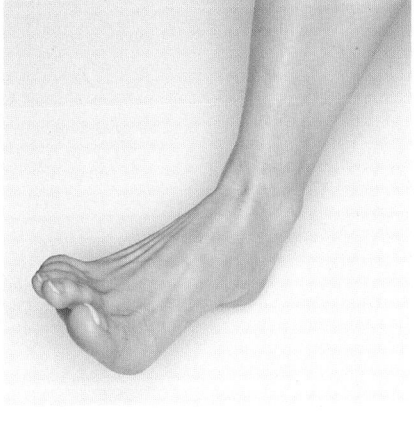

2 Flex the foot up and back, hold it there for a count of ten, and then relax. Repeat this ten times.

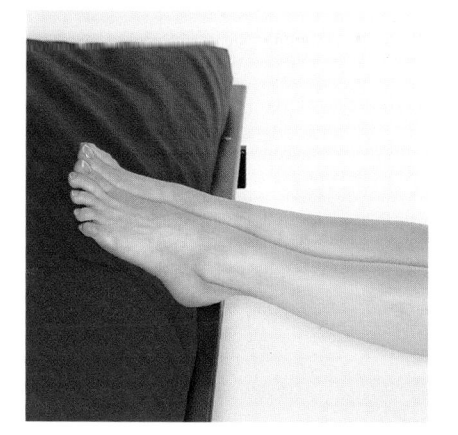

3 When you have finished exercising, lie flat on the floor with your feet raised.

LEG EXERCISES

What you need
Hard chair
Object such as
    wastepaper basket

The first of these exercises may be done anywhere there is a chair and a wastepaper basket. If you are using a woven wastepaper basket, like this one, be careful not to snag your stockings on it. Exercises 2 and 3 require a bit more room. Make sure that you have a comfortable floor or blanket to lie on before you start.

If you have goose-pimply legs and lifeless-looking, grey skin, rub your legs vigorously with body lotion every day before you begin your exercises. A massage with a body glove or loofah while you are in the bath or shower will help to prevent this by stimulating the circulation.

Make the most of your legs: everyone has a skirt length which they feel suits them best – mid-calf length skirts are flattering to most legs, but be careful that the hemline does not cut across the widest part of your calves. Similarly, heavy legs do not look their best in pale-colored stockings.

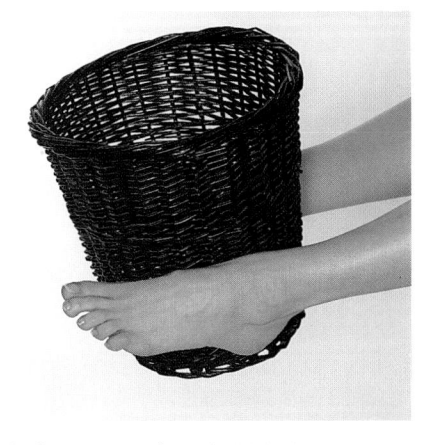

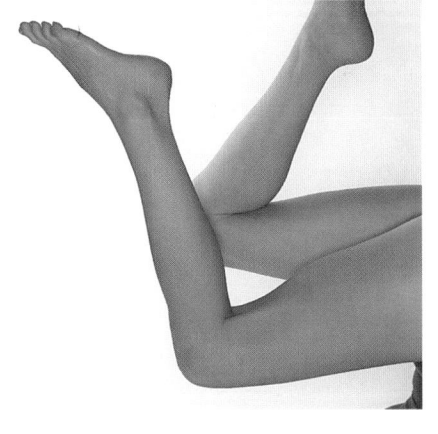

1 *Sitting on a chair, hold the basket between your ankles. Lift and hold for a count of twenty. Repeat ten times.*

2 *Lie on your back, and lift your legs in the air. Supporting your hips, make bicycling movements with your legs.*

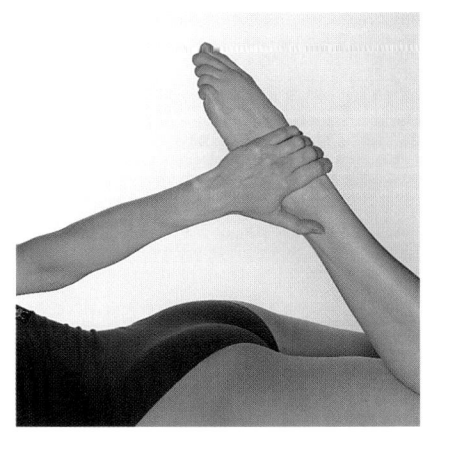

3 *Lie on your stomach and pull your ankle towards your bottom. Count to ten. Repeat twenty times and then change legs.*

INDEX